EMDR Essentials

EMDR Essentials

A Guide for Clients and Therapists

Barb Maiberger

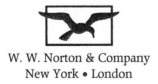

W. W. Norton & Company
New York • London

For information about permission to reproduce
selections from this book, write to
Permissions, W. W. Norton & Company, Inc.
500 Fifth Avenue, New York, NY 10110

For information about special discounts for bulk purchases,
please contact W. W. Norton Special Sales
at specialsales@wwnorton.com or 800-233-4830.

Composition and book design by Bytheway Publishing Services
Manufacturing by Haddon Craftsmen
Production Manager: Leeann Graham

Library of Congress Cataloging-in-Publication Data

Maiberger, Barb, 1961–
    EMDR essentials : a guide for clients and therapists /
Barb Maiberger.
        p.   cm.
Includes bibliographical references and index.
ISBN 978–0-393–70569-0 (pbk.)
1. Eye movement desensitization and reprocessing.   I. Title.

RC489.E98M35   2009
617.7'06–dc22   2008034579

ISBN 13: 978-0-393-70569-0 (pbk.)

W. W. Norton & Company, Inc., 500 Fifth Avenue,
New York, N.Y. 10110
www.wwnorton.com

W. W. Norton & Company Ltd., Castle House,
75/76 Wells Street, London W1T 3QT

1 2 3 4 5 6 7 8 9 0

Contents

PART II: TRANSFORMATIONAL STORIES

Acknowledgments

I want to thank all the people who have helped make this book possible. Thanks to Molly Gierasch for her expertise, guidance, and support, and for all the hours of reading and editing my book. I could not have done this without her.

Thanks to all my clients, who teach me about EMDR on a daily basis, and to those clients who generously shared their stories.

And thanks to all the therapists who come to me for EMDR consultation. They inspired me to write this book, and their excitement for the work keeps me growing as a therapist. Lauren Bouche for introducing me to EMDR and insisting that I would love it. To my colleagues, Stacey Arnett, Jonathan Williamson, and Dawn Deopardi, for their contributions to this book and for encouraging me to complete it. Zona Scheiner for giving me great professional advice and for being so generous with her time and knowledge.

To my wonderful friends Dori Jenks, Dotty Uhl, and Kelly LaValley for their encouragement, support, and love. Kelly Moye and Keith Warner for reading my book and giving me feedback. Rick Moss for his support, hours of brainstorming, and photos. Phil Penningroth for his creativity and vision that kept me on track at all times.

Finally, I would like to express my appreciation to Francine Shapiro for her dedication to developing EMDR and having the passion and drive to share her work with the world.

EMDR Essentials

Introduction: How I Came to Practice EMDR

My name is Barb Maiberger and I'm an eye movement desensitization and reprocessing (EMDR) consultant and therapist. You'll get to know more about me as you read along. Right now, though, I'd like to take a couple of moments to tell you about this book.

I decided to write *EMDR Essentials: A Guide for Clients and Therapists* because I believe in EMDR therapy and have found that many people either know nothing about it or have been badly misinformed. My purpose here is to tell you what I know in a simple, straightforward way. While there's some technical terminology that I think is important for you to understand, this is not a textbook or research tome (although there are some citations and references in the back for those who want to read more). I just want to tell you about EMDR so that if you or someone you care about ever needs therapy, you'll know more about what to expect and how to prepare yourself for treatment.

This is not a very long book. Really, it's a handbook, and should be a pretty fast read. It's organized in two parts for easy use and understanding. In Part I you will find an explanation of EMDR, the phases of EMDR treatment, the nature of trauma and its effect on memory, theories about why EMDR works, how EMDR can work for children, and EMDR safety issues. Part II illustrates all the information you read in Part I with inspirational stories about my clients, their issues, and how EMDR helped them.

Although there's a logic to the flow of chapters, the book has also been designed so that you can jump into any chapter and learn something important about trauma, EMDR therapy, how EMDR was discovered, and much more. Because of this design, if you do decide to read it from cover to cover, you'll find some repetition. That's because a lot of the most important information applies in different contexts. Sometimes you will see "she" used more than "he" because I have worked with more women over the years, but whatever I am saying throughout the book can apply to either gender.

The sole purpose of this book is to inform you, the client, about what to expect when you enter EMDR therapy and how it may help you heal from trauma. This book is NOT meant to teach therapists how to do EMDR therapy. Therapists must be trained in EMDR International Association–approved courses where they receive certificates proving that they have completed the basic EMDR training.

How I Came to Practice EMDR

When I began my career as a massage therapist, I loved helping people feel better. Some came to me for relaxation or to soothe aches and pains. Others came for treatment of traumatic injuries caused by automobile wrecks, other accidents, or illness. The more experienced I became, the more convinced I was that I could heal with my hands. But then something strange and unexpected happened. As I worked with people seeking just relaxation, some of them began to respond like victims of trauma. When I massaged a trauma victim, I had come to expect that some particular touch—I could never predict just what—might throw her back into the traumatic experience. Whenever that happened, she would respond with fear, anger, grief, or some other powerful emotion that would often take us both by surprise. Strong physical sensations would arise spontaneously in her body and she would begin to cry, cringe, or tremble. Sometimes a client would remember a trauma from childhood such as physical or sexual abuse. But often she (or he) did not remember anything and couldn't say why she was suddenly feeling such disturbing emotions and sensations. Puzzled, I spoke to other massage therapists and discovered that many shared my experience. It seemed that many people held forgotten yet troubling memories in the very muscles, sinews, bones, and cells of their bodies. My hands were evoking emotional and physical responses that as a massage therapist I wasn't trained to handle. The best I could do was to refer them for psychotherapy.

Frustrated by my own limitations and what I came to suspect were the limitations of traditional psychotherapy, I decided to study the mind as well as the body, and especially the connection between the two. Looking back, I realize now that this interest in what's called the body-mind connection began when I was a little girl. As a member of the Camp Fire Girls, I had to create an Indian name for myself that was a reflection of who I believed myself to be. The name that came to me was "Chee-Ron-Ta," a person who sees beauty in dance and happiness in giving. Little did I know that at that time I had chosen a name that reflects who I am today, a therapist who loves to dance.

I started dancing when I was 4 years old. I loved moving and how alive it made me feel. Dancing was my passion and I decided to major in dance in college, and received a bachelor of fine arts degree in modern dance. I performed professionally for several years. While in college I discovered massage therapy at a dance festival and I knew that when I stopped performing I would follow this career. While recovering from a dance injury, I studied massage therapy at the Swedish Institute of New York. There I learned how to read the body for habitual patterns and to help clients find new freedom in their bodies. I loved massage but came to realize that I needed to study psychology to understand what was happening to my clients when they would have emotional experiences on my massage table. I needed to understand on a deeper level how people experienced the physical and emotional effects of my work. How could a past, forgotten event remain so disturbing that fear, rage, grief, or some other emotion repeatedly disrupted a person's present life and negatively influenced how he lived—or, more often, how he failed to live?

I returned to graduate school and studied somatic psychology at the Naropa University in Boulder, Colorado. Somatic psychology is an interdisciplinary practice that focuses on the body. In contrast to a traditional talk therapist, a somatic psychotherapist first considers a client's postures and gestures, muscular patterns, chronic contractions and tensions, the range and shapes of movements, ways of breathing, skin color and tone, physical habits, use of space, and body pulsations and rhythms, as well as more subtle body energies, all as part of the therapy process.

Because I was particularly interested in trauma, I chose to do my counseling internship at the Boulder County Safehouse, a shelter for abused women. There I began to see the impact of traumatic abuse on the lives of women and their children, not just the obvious trauma of beatings but also how present trauma seemed to evoke more subtle, often forgotten traumas from childhood that caused them to see themselves in negative ways that led to destructive choices. As I watched women struggle to find the strength to overcome obstacles and rebuild their lives, I realized that many were suffering in ways I had never before recognized, and I came to appreciate the vagaries of the heart, the complexity of the soul, and how difficult it can be to heal. Certainly, I was often helpful to these women, but I still sensed there was something missing. I wanted to do more.

About that time, I heard a lecture at Naropa by Bessel van der Kolk, a world-renowned expert on the treatment of trauma. He spoke about a treatment called EMDR, or Eye Movement Desensitization and Reprocessing. This was the first time I'd heard about it and I was skeptical. Even though he showed some impressive before-and-after brain scans of people who had experienced EMDR, the therapy didn't seem body centered and other therapists I respected gave it mixed reviews. Because they misunderstood the basic neuropsychological principles involved (so I realized later), most considered it a variation of cognitive behavioral therapy, a type of talk therapy that was (and generally still is) the current dominant psychotherapeutic method for treating trauma. While a few considered it the wave of the future for the treatment of trauma, many others feared it worked too fast (if it worked at all) and could harm a client, or dismissed it as just another therapeutic fad that would soon fade away.

Several years passed. One day I was telling a colleague what I considered an amusing story. In those days I lived in a small town about 10 miles from Boulder and had to drive to work every day on a freeway that was heavily patrolled by the police. Every time I saw a police car, even if I wasn't speeding, I feared I was going to be stopped, maybe even arrested. With the fear came sweat, a racing heart, and shallow breathing. "See," I told my colleague, chuckling, "all I have to do is remember and it happens." Fortunately, she was not amused. Instead, she suggested, "You should try some EMDR."

"The eye thing? But why?"

"So you won't have to feel this way anymore."

"It's nothing, really."

"Nothing? Really?"

Suddenly, I thought about all of my clients who responded in the present as if they were reliving some past trauma. And if I was honest with myself, the fact that I could not recall any traumatic event did not mean that one did not exist. Still, I resisted. I felt nervous, uneasy. But when she offered a trial session to deal with this specific issue, how could I refuse?

This was my first experience with EMDR. Through the years I'd continued to hear mixed reviews and, though curious, I'd never bothered to learn any more about it. My colleague worked with me to resolve my fear and my physical responses to the sight of a police car or a policeman on the highway. Later, I'll describe the process of EMDR therapy in more detail. Here, however, let me simply share my experience.

As my therapist asked me questions to connect me to the fear and physical sensations of seeing policemen on the highway, I found myself suddenly remembering a time years before when a police officer pulled me over. He didn't tell me why, he just demanded my license and insurance. Standing beside the car in his uniform, a baton and gun hanging from his creaking leather belt, he seemed as huge and powerful as I felt tiny and insignificant. Petrified, I began to shake and sweat and in my panic and confusion gave him an expired insurance card, and then couldn't find the updated one. Also, I'd recently moved and my license plates had expired—the reason he'd pulled me over. Bad plates, bad insurance; what else could go wrong? As it turned out, nothing bad happened. Luckily, my driver's license listed my new address and when I explained all of the circumstances, the officer let me off with a warning to get new plates.

Here, then, was a past event I had forgotten yet continued to hold in my body-mind as a present traumatic experience. Each time I saw a police car on the highway, my body-mind responded in the present as it had in the past, with all the physical and emotional symptoms of panic. With the help of my therapist, using EMDR desensitization techniques we worked with the past event until I could recall it without any emotional or physical response. Still, I was skeptical and left my friend's office wondering how effective the treatment would prove in the real world. Driving home, I was disappointed not to see a police car. And then I pretty much forgot about the whole thing until a few days later, when a police car passed me on the highway and I hardly noticed—until I realized I'd felt no emotional or physical response. Then I was convinced that with the help of EMDR I was free of that past trauma.

Finally, I realized that EMDR was an integrative therapy that could offer something very special to my clients. I immediately signed up for Level 1 training through the EMDR Institute and by the end of the course had become such a convert that I couldn't wait to use it. Of course, EMDR isn't right for every client and I quickly learned that there's a difference between using EMDR and using it wisely. Accessing old trauma can be scary and emotionally upsetting, so it's important to assess when and how appropriate it is to use EMDR. Failure by a therapist to skillfully guide and facilitate the process from the beginning to the end can, indeed, cause harm. Also, inadequately trained therapists and therapists who skip steps to speed up the process, or fail to complete sessions, leave clients convinced that EMDR doesn't work. Such negative word of mouth discourages traumatized people from taking advantage of a therapy that can change their lives.

I decided to write this book to explain EMDR to people who might benefit from the therapy but know little about it or are skeptical of its benefits. Since its discovery in 1987, EMDR has grown in both theory and practice and has become a psychotherapeutic model for integrating the cognitive, emotional, and physical. After a decade of practice and training as a psychotherapist, I am now a certified EMDR therapist and an approved consultant through EMDRIA, the EMDR International Association. I also work with Molly Gierasch, PhD. She is an EMDRIA approved instructor of the basic EMDR trainings and I am now an instructor for those trainings. As therapists learn EMDR psychotherapy, instructors stress skills to help them work with clients so that their practice will be both thorough and safe.

In this book you will read what EMDR has been like for my clients. (I have changed their names and identifying details to protect their privacy.) As you read their stories, you will see how I track what is happening in their bodies and so access trauma in a way that often cannot be expressed in words. In fact, talking about it sometimes hurts; the therapeutic cliché "just let it all out" can do more harm than good, because retelling a traumatic story over and over actually entrenches the traumatic memory and its symptoms deeper into the body-mind. You will see that as a body-centered psychotherapist, I hold the belief that thoughts and feelings are expressed through the client's body-mind connection. This means that what people are thinking and feeling is expressed in how they move or don't move in the world, and these feelings and thoughts also have a profound effect on their emotional well-being. I will be exploring in later chapters how EMDR was developed and how it integrates many models of psychotherapy, including body-centered principles.

Perhaps like you, when many of my clients first heard about EMDR it seemed abstract and theoretical, and the thought of beginning therapy was scary (as it was for me) because it requires trust in the therapist and trust in an unfamiliar therapeutic process. It may take some letting go to do the work and discover if EMDR is right for you, but I am convinced it will be worth it. In my practice I have found that EMDR has helped 75% of my clients; for the other 25% I use other methods of treatment or refer to other therapists for specific types of work that I do not specialize in.

EMDR is not magic, but when it works, the relief is so great that it often feels magical. Here you will read what my clients experienced before, during, and after EMDR as they struggled to resolve issues in their lives, sometimes in a couple of 50-minute sessions, but usually over the course of several sessions. As you read, you will see that some changes can be quite dramatic and others very subtle. But in the end, one change is always the same: with the help of EMDR, people who have been burdened for years with trauma they often could not remember find that they no longer react the same way to present situations that before stimulated a psychological or physiological response in the body-mind and so now can live fully, free of the past. Of course, as with any therapy, it's your commitment to healing that makes the work possible. The path is not always an easy one but I believe that if you are willing to face the fear that is holding you back from the life you long to live, with the help of EMDR you can find a new way of being in the world. May this book be your first step on the path to healing.

PART I

An Inside Look
at EMDR Therapy

A journey of a thousand miles begins with a single step.

Lao-tzu

CHAPTER ONE

Beginning EMDR Therapy

The best way out is always through.

Robert Frost

Whenever I meet people and they ask, "What do you do, Barb?" I say, I help people feel more empowered through healing emotional pain. I'm a psychotherapist and I specialize in healing trauma through EMDR. EMD...what? EMDR: it stands for eye movement desensitization and reprocessing, a mouthful I don't expect you to remember. What I do hope you'll remember is that EMDR is a therapy that helps people relieve their pain and suffering caused by traumatic events that have hurt them and left them in a state of distress. It is a therapy intended to help people clear past traumas in order to feel more present, satisfied, and effective in their current lives.

I realize that the word *trauma* can be scary for many people. My intention is not to scare you, but to educate you about trauma, EMDR, and how you might benefit from it.

EMDR is an inclusive therapy that integrates different aspects of various psychotherapeutic traditions. The goal of this therapy is to empower people to feel, think, and behave in new and healthier ways.

Choosing therapy can be difficult. You may still feel a stigma surrounding therapy, or that there is something wrong with you if seek help for an emotional issue. The truth is, if you seek out therapy you are a brave person who is willing to admit that as human beings we all sometimes need help to navigate in this world and in our body-mind. Our bodies and our minds are not perfect machines and they don't always feel the way we want them to. There's nothing shameful about asking for help. On the contrary, it is a basic human need to know other human beings who can witness our pain and reflect back to us about our problems, joys, and successes. I hope that after reading this book, if you are considering EMDR therapy you will embrace that choice and know you are headed down a new and exciting path. It may sometimes be challenging but, believe me, it will be worth the effort.

The job of an EMDR therapist is to be your guide and help facilitate your journey to empowerment. I am always reminded of the power of the EMDR process whenever I offer a session. Recently, while taking an advanced EMDR workshop and sharing a hotel room with Gwen, a colleague of mine, in Vail, Colorado, I did some impromptu EMDR.

Gwen complained that she was becoming allergic to our hotel room as the days progressed and wondered how she was going to survive the rest of the workshop. I suggested that we try some EMDR, looking at her current symptoms and checking to see if there was any emotional trauma that was connected to how she was currently feeling. After all, we were at an EMDR conference and it seemed like the perfect opportunity to try EMDR with an issue I'd never worked on before. I had Gwen focus on her allergy symptoms—"itchy eyes, scratchy throat, coughing and congestion, and physically just feeling under the weather." I asked her, "What is the worst image that represents all of these symptoms for you?" She said, "I'm in the hotel room sneezing, all alone, curled up in a chair with a blanket over me." I then asked her, "When you think about this, what does this make you believe about yourself now?" She replied, "I can't make it." I then asked, "When you think about this image, what would you like to believe about yourself now?" She said, "I'm healthy and okay." I then asked her, "When you think about this image and the words 'I'm healthy and okay,' how true does that feel on a scale of 1 to 7, where 1 is false and 7 is completely true?" She replied, "2." I instructed her, "When you concentrate on being in the hotel room, alone and sick, with the words, 'I can't make it,' what emotions come up?" She said she was feeling "annoyed, frustrated, bad about feeling bad." "On a scale of 0 to 10, where 0 is no disturbance and 10 is the worst possible disturbance, what would you rate your feelings now?" She answered, "9." I asked her to notice where in her body she felt all these sensations and emotions. "In my face and head and all over my body—yuckiness all over." I asked her to trace this feeling back in time, without censoring, to see if any earlier memory would arise. After a time she said, "No, all I can feel is the yuckiness."

At this point, I started doing bilateral stimulation (I'll explain that later in the book). As she stayed with her feelings, different memories arose about when she was traveling a lot in her life and how difficult it was to travel. She said that she always had to "just make do" and not let others realize that she was having a hard time. Next, she remembered being back in grade school and going to the nurse's office. When she came back to her classroom, the teacher asked her a question that had been discussed while she was gone, and she didn't have the answer. Remembering, she said, "This is nonsense! The teacher set me up to feel bad about myself." Then she realized that, for her, this workshop was also nonsense and she said "I really don't want to be here and my body is telling me I really don't need to be here. I don't need to do this to myself anymore; I've studied enough."

At this point I had her refocus her attention on the first image of being in the hotel, alone and sick, and asked her what she noticed. She said, "I don't have to like Vail, or the values of the community. I'm not comfortable here and I don't have to be allergic to not like Vail." She stated that her symptoms had drastically lessened and she felt much better. I asked her, "When you think of the image now, how disturbing is it to you on a scale of 0 to 10, where 0 is no emotional disturbance and 10 is the worst?" She said, "0." I then asked her, "When you think of the image with the words, 'I'm healthy and I'm okay,' how true do those words feel now on a scale of 1 to 7 where 1 is completely false and 7 feels completely true?" She immediately said, "6." I added some bilateral stimulation to strengthen this belief and then checked in again. She noted that she now totally believed she was healthy and okay and rated herself a 7.

I then had her take this belief into the future, imagining staying in the hotel feeling healthy for the rest of the workshop. We continued with bilateral stimulation until she felt strongly that this could be true for her. I had her imagine the original issue with the words, "I'm healthy and I'm okay," and then scan her body for any residual body information. She said that the symptoms were 90% gone and she was more conscious about what her body was trying to tell her. Having her experience validated and not judging herself for having these feelings was a huge relief.

The following day Gwen said, "I feel so much better I can hardly believe it. My symptoms are barely present." As time passed, Gwen felt better and better. The processing was continuing on its own, a hallmark of EMDR. By understanding what she was truly feeling and not trying to "just make do" anymore, Gwen could let herself have a different experience and her body-mind was much happier. She actually enjoyed the workshop and felt she had gained some new helpful skills for EMDR therapy. I was once again excited that EMDR could make a difference in someone's life. This session may sound complicated, but I will go over it step by step throughout the book to help you understand the process of an EMDR session more fully.

Trauma and EMDR

Let's look at EMDR so that you can understand what it entails and how it can be helpful. When most people think about trauma, they think about rape, sexual abuse, auto accidents, and war. But Dr. Francine Shapiro, the developer of EMDR, defines trauma in a more inclusive way. Whenever something happens that you are unable to process and you are left feeling in distress, with symptoms that just won't go away, that's also considered a trauma response. She also says that memory is stored in the brain and that symptoms you experience may be felt throughout the body. I like to think of this in terms of the body-mind connection—that what we think and feel reflects our pains and joys through behavioral and thought patterns. As a body-centered psychotherapist, I believe that in order to heal you have to deal with the whole person, both the body and mind. If you think about it, you may discover that you've experienced a lot more trauma than you imagined. Most people have. If the trauma remains unresolved, it may be causing symptoms in your present life.

There are many kinds of symptoms or problems clients bring to therapy from home, work, or relationships. Here are some of the symptoms client have reported to me when entering therapy:

- Inability to be assertive
- Struggles with body image
- Feeling anxious or depressed most of the time
- Tendency to procrastinate
- Behaviors that sabotage their efforts
- A low tolerance for frustration or anger
- Difficulty concentrating
- Loss of interest in activities or goals
- Fights a lot and experiences a lot of anger
- Abuses substances (addictions)

- Struggles with making decisions
- Suicidal and self-abusive behaviors
- Somatic illnesses
- Sexual dysfunction
- Feelings of panic

If you are experiencing some of these symptoms, EMDR might be the answer for you. The symptoms can be an indication that a trauma or a memory of a past experience may exist, and you still need to deal with it.

EMDR is based on the premise that people inherently move toward health and given the opportunity, the brain knows how to heal on its own. Sometimes an event gets locked into our brain and for some reason can't integrate and become a normal, processed memory. Instead, when the event and all the emotions and sensations associated with it activate the past unprocessed memory from a present-day stimulus, the symptoms of the traumatic event appear, often with disturbing effect.

EMDR work consists of healing past traumatic events that haven't yet been integrated. EMDR helps facilitate activation of the brain's inherent information processing system to begin to do what it does naturally in order to help you find resolution of these stuck traumatic memories. Information in the form of memories is stored in memory networks that, when activated by the EMDR process, allow you to access related thoughts, images, emotions, and sensations. In this way you're able to work through and heal a past trauma relatively quickly, so that the present and future will no longer be linked to a dysfunctional past. This is considered the reprocessing of the traumatic event. Once that happens, you can let go of what I call the emotionally disturbing pieces that cause trauma symptoms and you can begin to transform your sense of self in relationship to the traumatic memory or, if they are present, positive aspects of the memory can naturally move to the forefront and become integrated.

How does this work? In an important sense, EMDR is a three-part treatment in that it deals simultaneously with the past, present, and future. Your therapist is your expert guide to facilitate this healing process. This includes a technique known as bilateral stimulation (BLS), which is used to activate the brain so that it can begin to process and integrate dysfunctional stored information—those locked traumatic memories—in a more adaptive way. You might see BLS called dual attention stimulation (DAS) or eye movement desensitization (EMS) in other texts. BLS is a disarmingly simple process that creates a powerful effect. It consists of an alternating left-right stimulation of the body and the brain. This is accomplished with eye movements, tones, music, hand pulsers, or sometimes touch. During BLS your therapist will ask you to focus on an internal state, usually a memory, an image, or a physical sensation, while the left and right sides of your body (and perhaps the left and right lobes of your brain) are externally stimulated in an alternating sequence. The speed and intensity of the stimulation can be varied depending on what feels right to you or seems most therapeutically effective to your therapist. The type used depends on the client's preferences. I have found in my own practice that all methods work and that each client has a favorite that works for him or her. Let's look more closely at each type of BLS so you can get a sense of what I am talking about.

Eye Movements

When EMDR was first discovered, Francine Shapiro used eye movements exclusively to facilitate the processing of trauma, and to this day only eye movements have been researched. If you choose to use eye movement, your therapist will sit across from you, slightly off to one side, so that you will be looking only at your therapist's hand or an object she is holding, such as a wand. Your therapist will put two fingers together and hold them directly in your line of sight and then move them back and forth in an even rhythm. You will be asked to hold your head still and just move your eyes back and forth as you follow your therapist's fingers. Your therapist will use a comfortable speed so that you will be able to track the fingers or object without any discomfort. Some therapists use a light bar to create the same effect. She will ask you to look at a machine and with your eyes follow a light that moves back and forth, right to left to right. When considering eye movement for BLS, be aware that this method is not recommended if you have any eye limitations or if you have a history of seizures, migraines, or head injuries.

Tac/Audio Scan

A Tac/Audio Scan is a small mechanical device connected by wires to two almond-shaped pulsers that you will hold, one in each hand. Many of my clients call these buzzers and one of my clients took to calling them her "buzzy bees." During BLS these pulsers will vibrate one at a time to provide alternating stimulation. These are vibrations and not electrical shocks. As with any of the BLS methods, the speed and intensity of the pulses can be changed to fit the needs of the client. Many clients find this device soothing, sometimes almost hypnotic. I use the Tac/Audio Scan produced by NeuroTek, a company in Colorado. Only EMDR-trained therapists can purchase these devices.

Tac/Audio Scans also have headphones to deliver bilateral audio tones or music from ear to ear. The speed and volume can be adjusted.

Some clients like to use the pulsers and the headphones at the same time.

Touch

Using touch for BLS, your therapist will tap on your hands or knees to create the alternating stimulation. I've found that some clients who feel sensitive about the other modalities prefer the comfort of human touch. However, if you have any history of physical abuse, this may not be a good option for you. If it still feels best to you, talk it over with your therapist to make certain that you're both in agreement and comfortable using touch to facilitate your processing.

BLS is considered the essential technique for EMDR sessions and is used in three different phases of EMDR treatment. First, during the preparation phase it helps build skills. When you add BLS to a positive feeling state, it becomes what in EMDR is called resource development installation (RDI). It can be used with any positive emotion or sensation to enhance the experience of relaxation, sense of well-being, or empowerment. Second, it's used when you process traumatic material in the desensitization phase. Finally, it is used when the client moves into the installation phase, where new thoughts and feelings are integrated and enhanced. I will be talking about all of the phases in detail later in the book. For now, however, just know that BLS powerfully facilitates the EMDR process and at the end of treatment your original traumatic event will no longer feel as vivid or disturbing and your trauma symptoms will be greatly relieved or will often have disappeared.

How to Find an EMDR Therapist

If you are considering EMDR therapy, how do you find an EMDR therapist and how will you know who is right for you? Here are some suggestions about where and how you can begin your search.

You can look at EMDRIA's Web site, www.emdria.org. Click on *About EMDR*. Scroll down and click on *Find a Therapist.* There you can provide information about where you live and search for a qualified therapist who belongs to EMDRIA in your area. EMDR therapists often have different levels of experience:

- EMDRIA consultants are licensed or certified therapists with a minimum of 3 years of experience in a field of psychotherapy who have completed an EMDRIA-approved

EMDR training program with a minimum of 300 EMDR
trauma sessions, have received consultation, and continue
to participate in EMDR education so that they stay current
in the field.

- EMDRIA certified clinicians are licensed or certified therapists
  with a minimum of 2 years experience in a field of psychotherapy who have completed an EMDRIA-approved EMDR
  training program with a minimum of 50 EMDR trauma sessions, have received consultation, and continue to participate
  in EMDR education so they stay current in the field.
- A member of EMDRIA is a licensed or registered therapist
  who has completed a EMDRIA-approved basic EMDR training and either has or is working toward completing a master's degree.
- A nonmember of EMDRIA is an EMDR therapist in your
  area who is not registered with EMDRIA but may have the
  qualifications to work with your trauma.

You can also look at the EMDR Institute's Web site,
www.emdr.com, and click on *Find an EMDR Clinician*. From
there you will enter the city in which you are looking for a
therapist and the qualified therapists' names will appear.

You can also ask friends who have experienced EMDR for a
referral. Therapists who don't do EMDR can usually refer you
to an EMDR specialist. Of course, EMDR therapists are often
listed under counseling or psychotherapy in your phone book
or on the Internet.

I believe that it's important to interview two or three therapists, so you can get a sense of how you feel with that person.
Research has consistently shown that one of the greatest factors in successful therapy of any kind is the relationship between therapist and client. When you meet a prospective therapist for the first time, notice how you feel when you are with
him or her. How do you feel in her space, and about how she
presents herself? It's important for you to get some sense of

how this person can help you with trauma symptoms such as emotions that feel overwhelming or behaviors that are sabotaging your goals. Even if you feel nervous, ask questions. In fact, if you're nervous, say so. The therapist will understand, and just expressing how you feel may lessen your anxiety. If you're concerned that you won't know what questions to ask, refer to the questions below before your interview, or take this book with you. Notice how the therapist answers your questions, and how you feel about what she says, and how she says it. Remember, your therapist is not your friend—she will be your expert guide, so pick someone you think and feel you can trust. Regardless of the professional qualifications, what is your gut feeling? Finding the right therapist is important, so you need to feel safe with and confident in the therapist who will act as your guide and facilitator in the healing process.

Here are nine sample questions that you can ask in your interview.

- Do you offer a free consultation so I can meet with you to see if EMDR is right for me?
- What is your level of training as an EMDR therapist?
- What is your background and training? Are you licensed?
- Have you ever worked with my issue (e.g., rape, depression, anxiety, auto accident) and had success with EMDR?
- How much EMDR do you practice on a regular basis?
- How long have you been practicing EMDR?
- What will our EMDR sessions look like?
- What do you charge for an EMDR session?
- How long are EMDR sessions?

Finally, and most important, once the interview is over take a moment of quiet time and ask yourself, How do I feel? Do I have a good feeling about our meeting? Remember, there are no right answers to these questions. But also remember that the relationship you develop with your therapist is one of the key components to successful therapy, so listen to your gut.

So I Found a Therapist—Now What?

You have just made a very important decision. The next step is the beginning of therapy. The fears you may have are natural. Your therapist will help you feel more comfortable by getting to know you better so she can assess how best to help you. This will also allow you to get to know her better, too.

I explain to clients that EMDR therapy can sometimes feel like a workout. At first, when you go to the gym it feels impossible to lift weights. You think you will never succeed. It's just too hard. Eventually, though, you begin to build muscle and the exercises get easier until one day you look at yourself and say, wow, I can do this! That's what trauma therapy is like. Through this work you will be building your emotional muscles. Therapy may seem intimidating at first, but as you learn what to expect and gain some experience you will begin to develop more skills and feel stronger and more confident. Before the first time you do EMDR you will have many questions, but after that first EMDR session you will feel how it works and will begin to trust the process that soon will bring change to your life. Eventually, most of my clients come in for their therapy session requesting to do EMDR.

Processing Trauma with EMDR

At this point I'm going to give you a simple explanation of EMDR. As you read the book, you will begin to understand it more deeply.

EMDR trauma work is designed to help you process a traumatic memory that for some reason did not get processed at the time it was experienced. This lack of processing could have happened for many reasons. Perhaps the event was just too overwhelming and you didn't know how to process it. Maybe there were too many things going on in your life and you couldn't handle one more thing. Or perhaps you were too young and might not have had enough support in your life to help you sort out the situation. You might habitually push things away that seem too painful. Whatever the reason, because you were unable to process this event, it got locked in your brain, with all the disturbing emotions and sensations that you originally experienced unchanged. Remembering this event, or even when you try not to remember because it's too painful, evokes trauma symptoms. You try to keep these memories at bay and might be successful for quite a while. But if a traumatic memory can't be processed when other events occur that remind you of the original traumatic event, emotions begin to emerge from the past memory network and connect to the present. You might try to protect yourself by putting it behind you—many people do—but eventually it takes less and less stimulus to activate the emotions associated with the traumatic memory. Often the feelings become so powerful that they can take over and leave you feeling out of control. When that happens it's like you've been hijacked by your emotions. Your reaction is not proportional to the present stimulus; some insignificant event can trigger an explosion. It's also not in direct relationship to the current moment, because the emotions of the past events feel as if the bad things are happening right now.

When something traumatic interrupts the natural progression of processing a memory, then memories of a traumatic event can get locked in their own neural network. Physical sensations, emotions, and thoughts associated with the traumatic event get locked up in a way that, without treatment, may lead to increasingly dysfunctional behavior or disturbing symptoms. EMDR is designed to help you identify and process these stuck traumatic memories so that you can be symptom free and more present and alive in your current life. When traumatic memories have been cleared and everything in your system is working efficiently, the brain can take in information, sort it accurately, and process it into long-term memory. At that point you will have learned what you needed to learn. You will still remember the traumatic event and will have a story to tell about it. But you will be able to remember and tell the story without the emotional charge that was so disturbing before EMDR.

When you begin to work with your trauma in therapy, something I tell my clients might be helpful to keep in mind. Processing trauma with EMDR is like traveling on a train from Colorado all the way to Maine. As you ride, you look out the train window and watch the scenery go by: rivers, roads, prairies, trees, clouds in the sky. It's the same with your trauma. As your therapist guides you to remember your trauma, the images, emotions, sensations, thoughts, and beliefs associated with that trauma will pass by in your body-mind. The therapy will light up the memories in your brain so that you can begin to process the traumatic event.

In order for the train to move, we have to start it by introducing bilateral stimulation. This alternating stimulation activates the brain in such a way that it begins to process the event in a way that wasn't possible before. The train will start and stop in different stations as you process the trauma. When the train starts, you will be using BLS and when the train stops, the BLS stops. You will know that you are in Maine when you can remember the traumatic event without any emotional disturbance. By the time you reach Maine, you will have found your way through the trauma and will feel more empowered and positive about yourself.

This is a wonderful part of the therapy because clients often feel such relief. I explain to my clients that we want the past to be in the past where it belongs. We are not going to erase the memory but we are going to change your relationship to the memory. We want it to become just a memory rather an active, living, fire-breathing story that is controlling your life from behind the scenes. The beautiful part of EMDR is that you get to keep the good parts of your memory and let go of the disturbing parts. You still may not like what happened, but after EMDR you won't be ruled by the event any longer. Your therapist will support you in this by helping you integrate new feelings, thinking, and behaviors into your daily life.

How Clients Describe the EMDR Process

How EMDR works and what it feels like can seem abstract until your first experience. Often new clients ask, what does EMDR feel like? It's an interesting question. Let me tell you first about my own experience. When my therapist sets up the session I can see an image and recognize the associated negative belief, emotions, and body sensations. Once the BLS begins, my process can be very sensory. I often just feel body sensations without any storyline. I might notice pain in my heart, or difficulty breathing, or heat in my hands, or my jaw clenching. I watch the moving sensations as if I'm seeing different notes played on an instrument. When the train stops, I report the sensations or whatever I'm noticing right in the moment. Sometimes new images arise to begin a story, or to offer a new insight. The process is never quite the same and it's surprising where it takes me. Although I'm always aware that I'm in my therapist's office and can sense her presence, I'm simultaneously in this very internal space within, witnessing a mystery unfolding.

My personal experience with EMDR has taught me that there is no way to know how traumatic memory will unfold and what a client will learn through the process. I've often asked my clients what processing trauma during that EMDR train ride feels like for them. To give you a preview of what you might expect, here are some of their unique and personal answers.

- "It is an internalized process where I released negative perceptions and then felt I could choose future responses that felt more supportive to me."
- "It's like a waking dream. Sitting with an image that evokes feelings and witnessing where those feelings are being felt in my body. The feelings sometimes bring up emotions,

memories, or just sensations in certain areas in my body. I stay in the waking dream until the feelings, sensations, or emotions pass and I arrive at the other side. The time that it takes to move through the dream is very quick and no words are needed to feel the relief. I've learned that avoiding going through the feeling or sensation is much harder than staying with it until it loses its charge. At that point the original discomfort no longer has the power over me that it did at the beginning of the EMDR session."

- "It's really powerful. It sounds kind of silly; you hold a little vibrating buzzer in each hand and they alternate vibrating back and forth. But it works. Somehow, you find yourself feeling different. Sometimes, you feel yourself feeling sad or angry or scared and you realize that you've been sitting on this feeling for years.... It's almost as if it was physically present in your body, like a dam or a hidden boil. Fully letting it out is very cathartic. Not only do you feel better, but you make room for holding something new and hopefully more satisfying—like joy or hope or a new sense of who you want to be."

- "At the start of sessions there is often discomfort, which can manifest emotionally and/or physically. There may arise a sense of mental discomfort, as well as a shakiness on the emotional level. Holding the pulsers, the healing begins immediately. There may be pain, tears, discomfort, but purging the charge is worth the travail."

- "The process felt difficult and due to the emotional pull, I felt resistance to continue—it felt too hard. With compassionate coaching from Barb and her encouragement to continue, I was able to finish with a feeling of subtle resolve. This does not mean I have forgotten the incident, but it allowed me to untangle from this emotional pull and to be able to recognize certain patterns in my childhood. I have come to realize my courage both then and now."

- "The process is primarily one of transforming negative

feelings into a more positive or accepting perspective. The hand pulsers are very soothing."

The Phases of EMDR?

EMDR is a process therapy. There are three roughly chronological phases to the treatment. Like all psychotherapies, EMDR therapy is both a science and an art. It is not, however, like following a recipe. Nor is it a magic one-session cure-all. What I'm about to tell you represents a guideline from which your therapist will probably work, although your process may not look exactly like this. Because you are a unique individual and your trauma is specific to you, your therapist is trained to work with you precisely where you are at any moment. Sometimes the phases of treatment may change order, or seem a bit different, or take more or less time than I describe here. Your therapist will make clinical decisions about your particular needs, pacing, and ability to integrate the work into your life. The setup may be modified depending on your issues or symptoms. Any modification will be designed to help facilitate what you need for successful EMDR therapy. It's vital in EMDR that you feel safe. Only then is it possible to set up a clear target and stimulate the memory network to process the trauma with BLS. Finally, it's important to end a session with safety measures so that you feel strong and can effectively live your life between sessions. You and your therapist will together discover what you need to make your therapy successful.

Let's look at the eight phases of EMDR therapy, so that you will know what to expect on your journey. I have divided the phases into two parts: laying the groundwork and EMDR trauma sessions.

Laying the Groundwork

Laying the groundwork is all about your therapist learning more about you so she can help prepare you to process any disturbing past experiences that may be creating dysfunction in your life. This occurs in the client history and preparation phases. As she learns who are, she will also help you to lay a solid foundation step by step, so that you can do safe and effective trauma work.

Phase 1: Client History

In this phase, your therapist begins by getting to know you better. Your therapist will take a thorough history of your life and begin to understand the symptoms, issues, and behaviors that are bothering you. Your therapist will note what traumas you have experienced in your life and what events have influenced who you are today. Your therapist will also look for your strengths and what brings you joy in your life. In this phase, you and your therapist will begin to identify trauma pieces to be worked on later with EMDR.

Phase 2: Preparation

In this phase, you and your therapist will begin to build trust. In addition, you will learn practical skills, how to feel stronger inside, and how to calm yourself through skill building. Your therapist will also explain EMDR therapy and what you can expect once you begin.

EMDR Trauma Sessions

There are 6 phases in the EMDR trauma sessions: (1) assessment, (2) desensitization, (3) installation, (4) body scan, (5) closure, and (6) re-evaluation. These phases progress in an order that safely achieves the best treatment. By this point, you and your therapist know which trauma (earlier disturbing event) will be addressed first. In this assessment phase the set up is the focus. Once that is completed, your therapist will facilitate the actual reprocessing of the traumatic event through the desensitization and installation phases. When appropriate, your therapist will guide you through a body scan to confirm that the trauma has been fully processed. All sessions end with a closure phase to make sure you feel safe and good about your work. Finally, all trauma work will be re-evaluated when you meet again with your therapist. This ensures that all reprocessing is complete.

Phase 3: Assessment

Next, you and your therapist will identify what EMDR therapists call targets. A target is the actual trauma, disturbing memory, or issue you will be working on. Your therapist will ask you a set of questions to clearly identify and assess the target. You will be guided to find the image, emotions, beliefs, and body sensations that are a part of that particular traumatic memory so that you will be ready for the next phase.

Phase 4: Desensitization

This phase is where the processing of the traumatic memory takes place. You will use a method of BLS to activate the brain to begin the reprocessing of the traumatic material. A scale is used in this phase to help you determine if the trauma has been completely processed.

Phase 5: Installation

In this phase, you will have processed the traumatic event and a more positive belief about yourself will naturally emerge. The focus of this phase is to concentrate on the full integration of a positive assessment of the new belief with the targeted incident or traumatic event. This new positive belief is then integrated with anticipated future events imagined and reinforced with BLS. A scale is used in this phase to rate how true this new belief feels to you. When the installation is complete the new belief feels completely true.

Phase 6: Body Scan

Your therapist will ask you to bring up the old image from the traumatic memory paired with the new positive self-belief, and will scan within the body for any residual tension, distress, or discomfort. If you have any remaining distress, you will continue to process with the BLS. If there is nothing left, you will proceed to the next phase.

Phase 7: Closure

Your therapist makes sure you are ready to leave your session and move on with your day, preparing you for what happens after EMDR sessions and making sure you are grounded and present.

Phase 8: Re-evaluation

In your next session you and your therapist assess if the work is complete for that piece of trauma or if there is more work to be done.

Each phase can take different lengths of time depending on the amount and intensity of the trauma you're dealing with and your support system. Once you have completed laying the groundwork, you will begin EMDR trauma sessions. You may alternate EMDR sessions with other types of therapy that will help you integrate the work until you feel it is complete. For some people, this whole process can take only a few sessions, while for others it can be a much longer process. How many sessions this takes depends on a number of variables. Allow me to repeat that EMDR is not a one-session therapy and is not a cure in the strict medical sense. Also, lay people should not attempt to practice EMDR on themselves. When a client works with a qualified therapist, however, EMDR is a proven, safe method to help work with and heal trauma and reduce or eliminate traumatic symptoms.

How EMDR Was Discovered

Now that you have a sense of EMDR therapy, let's take a look at how it was discovered. Like many effective treatments,

EMDR came about through a fortunate accident. However, as famous scientist Louis Pasteur once remarked, "In the field of observation, chance favors only the prepared mind." Pasteur knew what he was talking about. When he was experimenting to find a treatment for cholera, one of his assistants used a culture from an old jar to inoculate chickens. Instead of dying, the birds got sick and recovered, and when inoculated again didn't get sick at all. Thus was the principle of vaccination discovered. When Wilhelm Roentgen was experimenting with electrical discharges, he accidentally placed his hand between an electrical discharge tube and a screen coated with barium and, lo and behold, saw his bones through the shadow of his skin. This accidental discovery of X-rays won him the Nobel Prize. Bacteriologist Alexander Fleming spent countless hours cultivating bacteria in his laboratory. One day he noticed that a mold had invaded a petri dish—apparently it had floated in through an open window. When he saw under the microscope that bacteria touched by the mold were dying, he had the presence of mind to preserve what became the lifesaving drug penicillin.

I share these examples of what scientists call the principle of accidental sloppiness because, to my mind, Francine Shapiro's accidental discovery of EMDR is no less remarkable. In 1987 she was a graduate student studying psychology. At that time, she was experiencing some upsetting memories, thoughts, and emotions. One day while she was walking in a park, the upsetting thoughts and feelings suddenly disappeared. Surprised and relieved, but also puzzled, she consciously brought the memories, thoughts, and emotions back into her mind. To her amazement, she realized that they weren't as disturbing as they had been before. Most people would have been grateful and left it at that, but not Francine Shapiro. She wanted to know why. What could have effected this change? She reviewed in her mind what she'd been doing. She'd been upset . . . walking in the park . . . looking around . . . glancing from side to side. Walking in the park and looking around when she was upset were familiar. She'd done it many times before and experienced no relief. But glancing from side to side? Curious, she began to experiment. She observed that when she moved her eyes rapidly back and forth, left to right, disturbing memories and thoughts seemed to lose their emotional charge. Why? She didn't know. But because it gave her such relief, she continued her self-experiment until she became convinced that she might be onto something important.

Being a scientist, Dr. Shapiro proceeded to experiment on her friends and colleagues and found that what she'd discovered worked for them, too. She asked them to think of something disturbing and had them rapidly move their eyes back and forth. When some of them found it difficult to coordinate this rapid eye movement, she had people follow her finger as she moved it back and forth in front of their eyes. She experimented with the speed and direction of the eye movement to see what would prove the most effective. She also experimented with questions designed to help people connect more deeply and completely with their disturbing memories. Eventually this process developed into what Shapiro called EMD, or eye movement desensitization.

Positive results with her friends and colleagues encouraged Shapiro to try EMD with people who suffered from post-traumatic stress disorder (PTSD). She knew that a person may develop PTSD if he or she has been exposed to or witnessed a traumatic event in which there is an actual threat of death, serious injury, or harm to the self or others, or if he or she felt intense fear, helplessness, or horror. Such an event, experienced as overwhelming at the time, may continue to haunt people in the present. People suffering from PTSD often experience disturbing memories, thoughts, dreams, or nightmares. They may have trouble sleeping, feel irritable or angry, have problems concentrating, and remain hypervigilant, as they constantly guard against anticipated danger. Sometimes, triggered by an outside event that reminds them of past trauma, they feel as if the traumatic event is actually happening again—the flashback experienced by many veterans of combat. People who suffer from PTSD often interpret normal life stressors as life-threatening, and their survival response—fight, flight or freeze—is often so fast and unconscious that it's impossible for them to distinguish between the real threat that occurred in the past and the reality that there is no threat in the present. Needless to say, any of these symptoms can wreak havoc on life and relationships.

To expand her knowledge and understanding of what she'd discovered, Francine Shapiro arranged to do a research study with 22 people who suffered from PTSD. Her subjects included people who had been raped or sexually abused, and Vietnam War veterans who had never recovered from combat. She divided them into two groups. Each had one treatment session. In the control group, subjects were encouraged to do what therapists at the time thought was most therapeutic, that is, to remember and talk about the traumatic event in as much detail as possible. This group received no EMD. The other group was also encouraged to remember the traumatic event but did so while they received EMD. After the sessions, the EMD group reported that their symptoms felt less severe and that their anxiety had decreased. The control group felt little or no change. (For ethical reasons, the control group later received one EMD session.) When Shapiro checked in with her subjects between 1 and 3 months later, they reported positive behavior changes as well. The decrease in their symptoms and anxiety had empowered them to live more functional lives. After they received an EMD session, the controls reported similar changes (Shapiro, 1989a).

Simple and small as it was, Dr. Shapiro's research study put EMD on the therapeutic map. Years later, this study was replicated by three other EMDR therapists. The basic research design remained the same, but the second study included 40 men and 40 women who suffered from PTSD. They were randomly divided into two groups. One group received three treatment sessions, while the other group received no treatment (but did later, after the study was completed). This time both groups took a pretest to measure the level of disturbance caused by their symptoms, and then a post-test to assess the effect of the treatment. After treatment, the symptoms of those who had received EMDR had notably decreased, an improvement that continued when measured 15 months later. Members of the control group showed no improvement until later they, too, received EMDR (Wilson, Becker, & Tinker, 1997).

Meanwhile, Shapiro kept refining her methods. In 1990 she realized that the name EMD no longer fully described the therapy. That's when EMD became EMDR. She added the word reprocessing in order to explain another phenomenon she'd observed. As she used EMD to treat trauma, negative and disturbing images, beliefs, emotions, and sensations, clients' dysfunctional lives shifted and transformed and became more functional. She called this adaptive information processing (AIP). She believes that this is an innate neurological process that is jump-started by EMDR, allowing a person to move toward health. This internal system is intrinsic to everyone and that memories are stored in memory networks linked through associations based on perception. Memory networks are the gestalt or the whole of an experience through images, emotions, beliefs, and body sensations. Networks link together through the brain through associations. We'll look at this more closely in Chapter 2. When something happens that is difficult for a person to process, the information gets stored differently in the brain, which doesn't allow the information to connect with the AIP networks. Positive information or memories are also stored in memory networks. When the processing of EMDR begins, the unprocessed information starts linking through the AIP and transforms all aspects of the memory.

The other important piece of the AIP system is that when processing allows you to let go of the parts that are dysfunctional, you still get to keep the good parts. The memory does not go away—it is not like you go in with an eraser and it's gone forever. Rather, the brain releases or processes the disturbing aspects—whatever causes your traumatic symptoms—but the memory of the event along with your changed perspective on the experience remains. What EMDR helps you process are the disturbing images, beliefs, emotions, and body sensations that hold so much energy or charge that they disrupt your life. When these are processed or integrated, your distressing symptoms diminish or disappear. Through the process of EMDR therapy you become less agitated about a traumatic event and more an objective witness who can stand back and remember without the distress you felt before. Usually, this leads to compassion for yourself and others. Speaking personally, through my own EMDR experiences I have found a new ability to see others who have hurt me through different eyes. I have felt a deepening compassion for others' suffering and at the same time for my own so that I can move on in a way that's more clear and free. Yes, I realize that all of this may be hard to believe, but often something happens during EMDR that can be quite beautiful and, for some, even spiritual. When traumatic energy that has been held for so long is moved through the body and released, it creates a new sense of freedom. When this happens, your own truth arises naturally, along with a greater sense of clarity. It's as if a veil is lifted to reveal your true essence that you sensed was there but could never quite see. When this happens for clients, I feel blessed to be able to witness this revelation.

In the 20 years since Dr. Shapiro's remarkable discovery, EMDR has become one of the most researched psychotherapeutic treatments for PTSD, research that continues to expand into the treatment of other trauma. In 1995 the EMDR International Association (EMDRIA) was founded, a nonprofit organization dedicated to setting the standards for EMDR and offering programs to certify EMDR therapists and approved consultants. It also encourages research and provides ongoing professional support and education. While research (including the use of brain scans and other neurological technology) will increase understanding about how EMDR works, and education and training will improve the quality and ability of therapists, in the meantime you can be confident in the efficacy of EMDR, a treatment now recognized around the world that began when an upset psychologist with a prepared mind took a walk in the park.

CHAPTER TWO

Trauma, Memory, and Your Brain

We must always change, renew, rejuvenate ourselves; otherwise we harden.

Johann Wolfgang von Goethe

What is trauma? The short answer is: extreme stress. The longer answer is that trauma is any past experience that you perceive as negative and that negatively affects your present life. Trauma therapists often identify trauma as one of two types: big-T trauma or little-t trauma. Big-T trauma refers to trauma caused by an event that you perceived as horrific, unpreventable, and threatening to either your survival or the survival of others. Shocking, dramatic, and intense, these are often life-and-death experiences such as combat, rape, sexual abuse, criminal violence, a sudden accident, a natural disaster, or an unexpected loss. All trauma manifests in physical, sexual, or psychological symptoms. This kind of trauma is the easiest to understand for most people. Little-t trauma occurs when something happens to you that you are unable to process for any reason, whether the event seems large or small, which leaves you feeling in distress, leading to symptoms that interfere with your life. The effects can be long lasting and distort your perceptions of yourself and the world, damaging your self-confidence and your ability to engage positively and effectively in your daily life and your relationships.

Whether you suffer from big-T or little-t, the traumatic events involved are always real. The personal experience of trauma, however, is a matter of perception. We filter what we experience through our senses. Your reality is based on how you perceive a traumatic experience, and then what meaning it has for you. First, you hear, see, smell, taste, and feel an event. Then you think and feel about it. Carefree, crossing a street, you watch, horror-struck and paralyzed with fear, as a speeding car bears down on you and at the last instant, tires screeching, swerves aside. Later, you think, *I almost died.* You feel anxiety and you tell yourself that you were careless, stupidly reckless, and this, then, becomes the meaning associated with the trauma. The meaning you place on the traumatic event becomes superimposed on other aspects of your everyday life. Convinced that you're careless, stupid, and reckless, you become cautious, even fearful, and find it more and more difficult to cross a street, and panic when one of your children even approaches a curb. You're experiencing PTSD or a traumatic stress reaction. You've brought a past traumatic event into the present and it's distorting your perception of current reality and affecting your present ability to function. Because a traumatized person senses and feels the past experience as if it's happening now, you may not be able to recognize that there is no real danger. Or you may realize that there is no danger, but because there's a disconnect between your reason and your body-mind, you just can't help feeling and sensing that there's a threat. Just how and why EMDR therapists believe that this happens, I'll tell you when we discuss memory.

Symptoms of Trauma

People suffering from traumatic stress usually flip back and forth between what's called hyperarousal—being constantly on alert—and avoidance. While every person's situation is different, the following list will give you some idea of the symptoms often associated with hyperarousal and avoidance. Hyperarousal causes:

- Difficulty concentrating
- Sleep problems (difficulty falling or staying asleep)
- Hypervigilance (feeling constantly on guard)
- Overreacting to noises or other environmental cues that didn't bother you before
- Irritabity, anger, and outbursts
- Nightmares
- Recurrent and intrusive thoughts about the traumatic event
- Acting or feeling as if the experience is happening again in the present
- Intense psychological distress or physiological arousal when exposed to (internal or external) stimuli that symbolize or resemble an aspect of the traumatic event
- Flashbacks (suddenly feeling as though the event is happening in the present)

Avoidance causes:

- Sleep problems; difficulty falling or staying asleep (often to avoid nightmares associated with the event)
- Attempts to avoid thoughts or feelings associated with the traumatic event
- Attempts to avoid activities or situations that evoke memories of the traumatic event
- Inability to recall an important aspect of the traumatic event
- Feeling detached or estranged from others and your daily life
- A sense that you're unable to feel as you once did; you feel numb or spaced out, unable to care or to love
- Feeling less interest and pleasure in activities
- A sense of foreboding; anticipating a limited future, you

don't expect to have a career, marriage, children, or a long
life

As represented by any of these symptoms, a reaction to trauma
is a very troubling and trying experience, as you well know if
it has happened to you or someone you love. It's especially
disconcerting because it's so obvious that not everyone who
experiences a traumatic event ends up traumatized. Another
person terrorized by the same near-accident described above
might just shake it off and experience no traumatic aftereffects, just as many soldiers returning from combat never suffer from PTSD.

Why is this? The short answer is, no one knows for sure.
However, based on the experience of EMDR therapists and
other professionals who work with trauma, what we do know
is that the following factors may play a role in whether or not
a traumatic event later devolves into trauma:

- A prior history of trauma
- The degree to which any prior trauma was resolved
- Your family's history of coping with trauma and whether
  you learned to ask for help, to talk about your thoughts
  and feelings
- Gender
- Personality
- Age
- Your preferred choice of defense mechanisms
- The availability or absence of a good support system
- The intensity of the traumatic event
- Your individual genetic emotional makeup

Basic Structure of the Brain

Let's consider the brain for a moment. All species of living
things have a brain stem, the most primitive part of the brain.
Its job is to regulate the basic functions of life—breathing and
other metabolic processes—without our conscious awareness.

The brain stem is preprogrammed, so to speak, and does not have a capacity for learning.

The midbrain, or limbic brain, is the area where learning, memory, and emotions take place. The amygdala and the hippocampus are a part of this structure. The midbrain receives all information perceived by the senses and can compare past with present experiences.

The neocortex, or the thinking brain, is the latest evolutionary development and makes humans human. This is the executive part of the brain, which gives us the ability to have rational thought, even to think about thinking and feel about our feelings.

Threat and Stress

To understand why these factors affect whether or not a traumatic event is later experienced as trauma, it's important to know something about stress. The word *stress* is short for *distress* and derives from a Latin word that means "to draw or pull apart"; the Latin *districtia* literally describes "being torn asunder." If you've ever felt extreme stress, you can probably relate. It's also important to understand something about how stress affects the brain, and how chemical changes in the brain affect memory. This is a complex subject, so I'll summarize the essentials of what scientists think is happening in the brain.

When you (or another animal) are threatened, you respond in one of three instinctual ways: you run, you attack, or you're paralyzed by fear. But no matter whether you fight, flee, or freeze, your sympathetic nervous system (SNS) responds instantly to threat through your limbic system. In terms of human evolution, the limbic system is one of the oldest parts of your brain. The amygdala, a small, almond-shaped part of the brain located in the temporal lobe, is an important part of the limbic system. It assesses and stores information nonverbally. It has no capacity for language because there's no need to speak or understand words when you're a chimpanzee about to be devoured by a python, or a hominid about to be attacked by a lion on the African savanna, or an office secretary about to be humiliated by her boss. The limbic system has been with humans since the beginning and it's the amygdala that first, and instantly, decides if something threatens your survival. Before you're able to cognitively process the threatening situation in the prefrontal lobe of your brain, which is responsible for rational thought—literally, before you're consciously aware of what's happening—the amygdala has gathered information from your senses: sound, smell, taste, sight, and touch, as well as your body's position in space. It then "decides" if there's a threat and what you'll do about it: fight, flee, or freeze. I put "decide" in quotation marks because when we use that word we usually mean to make a conscious decision based on thought. Here, there's no thought involved. The amygdala's decision is based on a pure, unadulterated emotion: fear.

Joseph LeDoux, a neuroscientist at the Center for Neural Science at New York University, was the first to discover the role of the amygdala. His research showed how the amygdala can activate the nervous system before the neocortex has time to make a decision about the validity of emotion; for example, fight or flight. In one sense it can be said that our emotions have a mind of their own, including the amygdala, that is independent of the rational mind. In the face of environmental stimuli, the amygdala scans memory instantly for past experiences. If one key element of a present event is similar to a past traumatic event, for the amygdala that's a match, and it activates the nervous system. The brain's damper switch is in the neocortex, that part of the brain designed to assess the degree of threat so that we can deal with it more effectively. However, because the neocortex is slower to react than the amygdala, the nervous system can be triggered by the memory of a past traumatic event. In that event, the rational mind floods with emotion, making it hard to think straight.

If the amygdala decides that there's a threat, it secretes what are known as stress hormones to prepare the body to fight, flee, or freeze. If you've been in a similar situation before, a pattern has already been created that helps you—that is, your amygdala—interpret the threat. If you've previously hunted lions or you have to work with a nasty boss, your experience has taught you to recognize warning signs. If this is a new situation, the patterning begins now. Hunting lions or dealing with your boss in the future, you'll never forget this first attack. But always there will be a behavioral response; your body will move toward or away from the threat or get very still. Even if in a split second you realize that there is no threat—the lion is really just a house cat—your body-mind will already have reacted to protect you. The greater the threat, the stronger the arousal of the amygdala and the rest of the limbic system, and—this is very important—the more powerfully the experience will imprint in your memory.

Once the amygdala decides that there's danger, that information is passed on to the hippocampus, a small seahorse-shaped structure that's also an important part of the limbic system. "Passed on" really doesn't do justice to the speed of this process; it's so fast that, again, you're not consciously aware it's happening. All you know is that something feels scary out there.

The hippocampus then assesses and categorizes the incoming stimuli in a less emotional way. Do you recall a similar event? What, exactly, is it that you're sensing? Are there concepts and words to describe it—lion, house cat? Big lion? Lion cub? If your hippocampus categorizes what you're sensing as a threat, then it commands the release of the hormone adrenaline from your adrenal glands. The word *hormone* is derived from a Greek word that means, appropriately enough, "to set in motion." And that's exactly what adrenaline does; one way or another, in the interest of survival, your body-mind is set in motion. Your heart begins to race, your blood pressure goes up, your breathing gets fast and shallow, you sweat, your body odor may change (the smell of fear), and your digestion shuts down as blood is shunted to your fighting and fleeing muscles. Assuming that the lion hasn't yet attacked, if you're that hunter you get set to throw your spear, or take off for the tallest tree, or hunker down in the weeds and hope the big cat just ate.

Once the threat has passed, your parasympathetic nervous system (PNS) is supposed to take over and calm you down. Usually it does. But sometimes it doesn't, especially if the stress continues or increases in intensity. In the brain, the SNS fight-flight-freeze response always takes precedence over the PNS relaxation response. If you perceive that the threat continues—if you're hiding in the weeds from the lion—the hypothalamus then releases steroid hormones commonly know as corticosteroids, or cortisol. The trouble with cortisol is that while it may help you to survive the immediate threat, it also remains in your body and brain much longer than adrenaline and continues to affect and even damage brain cells. Some of these cells have to do with storing and retrieving memory. It also interferes with the function of neurotransmitters, the chemicals that brain cells use to communicate with each other. Too much cortisol can make it difficult to think and to recall long-term memories. That's why in a severe crisis you may feel and act befuddled. Your mind goes blank and you can't remember what you've been taught about lions because, in a neurological sense, "the lines are down."

Of course, not all news about stress is bad. A certain level of modulated stress actually increases your ability to learn. Some studies have found that when you relieve stress, your hippocampus can recover and begin to form new neuron cells. Also, as I mentioned before, several factors may play a role in whether or not a traumatic event later becomes trauma. Some of these are obvious, such as constant stress or the failure to learn coping skills as a child. Rigid psychological defenses or an absence of a good support system may make you more vulnerable. It also appears that the more intense the traumatic event, the more likely it is that you'll develop trauma. Gender, too, plays a role, potentially in a helpful way if you're a woman. Instead of fighting or fleeing, in response to stress many women "tend and befriend." Tending means caring for others, especially children, and befriending means social interactions such as talking on the phone with a friend. Researcher Shelly E. Taylor (Taylor, 2000) has observed, "The tend-and-befriend pattern exhibited by women probably evolved through natural selection. Thousands of generations ago, fleeing or fighting in stressful situations was not a good option for a female who was pregnant or taking care of offspring, and women who developed and maintained social alliances were better able to care for multiple offspring in stressful times." There's also a neurobiological explanation. Oxytocin is a hormone secreted in both men and women as a response to stress that's been shown to calm rats and humans, making them less anxious and more social. Both men and women secrete oxytocin, but male hormones seem to reduce the calming effect while the female hormone estrogen amplifies it. This difference in how men and women respond to stress may also be why women tend to live on average 7 years longer than men.

Stress Hormones and Memory

Stress hormones divert blood glucose to muscles (so you can fight or flee) and diminish the amount of glucose—energy—that reaches the hippocampus. Because the hippocampus also plays a vital role in learning and creating memory, when cortisol prevents enough glucose energy from reaching the hippocampus, its ability to learn and create new memories is compromised. Animal studies support this observation. Rats were stressed by an electrical shock and then put through a maze with which they were already familiar. When they were shocked either 4 hours before or 2 minutes before navigating the maze, the rats had no problem. But when they were stressed by a shock 30 minutes before, the rats were unable to remember their way through the maze. Why? Because the level of cortisol affects memory, and rat blood cortisol levels induced by stress were highest 30 minutes after the shock. Imagine the effect on memory of cortisol levels in a soldier during extended combat, or a woman being beaten and raped, or a child in constant fear of being emotionally or physically abused.

High and sustained cortisol levels may be one reason why some people can't remember a traumatic event. It also may be why short-term memory and learning are often the first casualties of a lifetime of stress. Another animal research study found that rats that were continuously stressed explored their surroundings as if they had sustained damage to their hippocampus; they showed no ability to learn or retain memories about where they were living. Among other brain researchers, Robert M. Sapolsky (1990) has shown that the longer and more often you experience stress that results in the secretion of cortisol, the more likely it is that your hippocampus will suffer some damage (Sapolsky, 1990). This is a problem because it's the hippocampus that tells the hypothalamus to shut off the cortisol. If the cells of the hippocampus are damaged by repeated stress, then it can't communicate as effectively with the hypothalamus. When that happens, you can't fully relax and you remain hyperaroused.

Now that we've considered rats, let's take a closer look at humans. How and why does the stress of a traumatic event devolve into PTSD? We know that continued high levels of cortisol can cause damage in pretty much anyone's hippocampus. However, research suggests that in a person who is suffering from traumatic stress, the ability of the hippocampus to categorize threat has fallen apart and the neurotransmitter connection between the amygdala and the hippocampus has been disrupted. Without an ability to categorize the threat—to take a moment to understand more about what's going on and further assess how dangerous it may be—you'll simply react. Without the mediation of conscious thought or language, the memory of the threat is stored in the amgydala as pure sensation and emotion—what you saw, heard, smelled, tasted, and felt, and the position of your body in space.

Bessel van der Kolk, director of the Trauma Center at Human Resources Institute Hospital in Brookline, Massachusetts, and an expert in the field of trauma and memory, conducted a study about the effect of EMDR in the treatment of trauma. In this study, he took SPECT scans (single photon emission computed tomography) before and after a sequence of three EMDR sessions. The pictures show activity in the brain, differing in brightness, color, and intensity. Although this is considered preliminary research (only 6 subjects and no control group), these findings suggest that the limbic arousal is overridden by the cortex with its new processed memory, thereby allowing a traumatized person to differentiate between an actual threat and a threat perceived only in memory after EMDR processing (Bergmann, 1998).

When a traumatic event devolves into a trauma reaction, the symptoms are a manifestation of the original stress and also add to the present stress. For example, the stress of trauma may contribute to flashbacks, but then the negative effect of flashbacks on you and your life and relationships adds more stress. Also, studies have shown that your nervous system will respond much faster to disturbing images than to pleasant and neutral images. You may do your best to forget a traumatic event, but when an image (and probably a thought or emotion) associated with it comes to mind, your nervous system will respond even before your conscious mind is aware of the image. Even if you don't realize it (probably because by now it feels natural), if you're suffering from trauma you are under constant stress.

Devolving Into Trauma

Now that you understand more about how stress, including stress caused by trauma, affects the body-mind, let's consider what happens when a traumatic event turns into a traumatic stress reaction. Remember, the ability to integrate a traumatic event without later symptoms emerging depends on your ability and willingness to remember what happened, as well as what the experience comes to mean to you. When we talk about a traumatic event, we often say that it was so overwhelming and scary that at the time we just couldn't process it. But what does that mean? At present, the best hypothesis (an educated guess that can be tested scientifically) is that when confronted with a traumatic event the brain is overwhelmed with information in the form of images, emotions, physical sensations, smells, and sounds. As we've seen, this causes immediate and severe stress. Stress causes a neurochemical cascade that can disrupt the normal processing of information by compromising the hippocampus and disrupting the connection between the hippocampus and the amygdala. When that happens, what's remembered remains in the amygdala as fragments of memory in their original distressing—"pulled apart"—state.

Scientists now know that memories are not stored in one specific area of the brain. Indeed, it appears that the same memory is stored in many different parts of the brain, depending on how different stimuli were perceived. So are different fragments of the same memory. Visual images are stored in the visual cortex, sounds in the auditory association area of the temporal lobe, smells in the olfactory cortex, thoughts in the prefrontal cortex, emotions in the amygdala, and so forth. These spread-out memories are linked through what EMDR therapists describe as a memory network. Memory networks are memories that have been linked in the brain through association. The associated memories can be thoughts, emotions, or sensory perceptions. The networks are like a spiderweb with almost infinite strands and connections. When something happens that affects your body-mind, it's as if something has touched the web. Tremors in the form of electrical and chemical neurotransmitters speed throughout your brain. If what you've perceived is novel, then your brain may form a new and discrete memory. (Just what you will remember depends on a number of variables that we don't need to consider here.) Most of the time, however, you will be reminded of something else (consciously, subliminally, or unconsciously) by whatever is happening. This will link the present experience by association to previous memories. According to Francine Shapiro, when a person is traumatized, thoughts, memories, images, emotions, and sensations related to the traumatic event are linked together and stored through these associations. However, because the damaged hippocampus has failed to categorize them, they remain as memory fragments in the amygdala in their original distressing state (Shapiro, 2001).

For example, the survivor of a car accident may retain disturbing memory fragments of her most recent experience stored together with similar disturbing memories from an earlier car accident. Later, recall of the recent event (say, the sound of squealing brakes) may trigger associated memories of a past event (shattering glass, blood, pain). This can happen even in situations where you have no recollection of the past traumatic event. If you haven't been able to integrate a traumatic event into your life, then one or more of these memory fragments can be triggered at any time, and apparently for no reason. You hear a noise and break out in an anxious sweat. Why, you wonder? The noise was no big thing. Some triggers are even subliminal; you see or hear but don't know you've seen or heard, but your body-mind still reacts. Without your conscious awareness, when a present stimulus triggers one of those disturbing memory fragments, it has the power to evoke symptoms of trauma.

As an EMDR therapist, I know that when you forget a traumatic event (either choose not to remember, or literally cannot remember) then your experience has failed to process. This is a shorthand metaphor that I often use to explain that the memory of a traumatic event has not yet been integrated. A number of scientists now believe that sleep plays an important role in the formation of memory, and that many short-term memories deemed important enough to remember are transferred into long-term memory while you sleep, probably during rapid eye movement (REM) sleep, when you're dreaming. Of course, not everything in your short-term memory is transferred into your long-term memory. You can, of course, choose to consciously remember something you feel is really important, but most of what you experience during a day isn't important enough to remember long term. When you sleep, your brain makes these decisions for you, so to speak. How and why does the brain choose to remember some things and not others? No one knows for certain, although observation suggests that you are more likely to remember something that carries some emotional resonance than, say, what you ate for lunch. A traumatic event that hasn't been processed always carries emotional resonance. If circumstances permit—if your hippocampus is not overloaded and can communicate effectively with your amygdala—the details of the event will be categorized and stored in your long-term memory as a coherent memory. In that case, you will be able to recall the memory without a trauma reaction. However, if circumstances were such that your memory system broke down and your long-term memories of the traumatic event now consist of only fragments in their original disturbing state, then ordinary events in your everyday life may trigger memories of this unprocessed trauma (and perhaps other associated traumas). When this happens, you will experience symptoms of trauma that disrupt your life and relationships, symptoms that you can no longer hold at bay.

Am I Suffering From PTSD?

In the 1970s, researchers started looking at combat survivors from the Vietnam War and came up with the formal diagnosis of post-traumatic stress disorder. This information became critical in understanding trauma and how it affects people's memories. PTSD is now a valid diagnosis for traumatized men and women who suffer the same symptoms when something horrible happens in their life. According to the *Diagnostic and Statistical Manual of Mental Disorders* (*DSM-IV*; American Psychiatric Association, 1994), PTSD is "the development of characteristic symptoms following exposure to an extreme traumatic stressor involving direct personal experience of an event that involves actual or threatened death or serious injury, or other threat to one's physical integrity; or witnessing an event that involves death, injury, or a threat to the physical integrity of another person; or learning about expected or violent death, serious harm, or threat of death or injury experienced by a family member or other close associate" (p. 424).

If you are suffering from trauma or feel stuck when trying to change destructive patterns of thought or behavior, EMDR might be right for you. Research shows that EMDR is an effective treatment for a variety of people suffering from the effects of many kinds of traumatic situations. Remember that trauma is defined by the experience of the individual and not necessarily just by the event. The following examples, taken from Francine Shapiro's book *EMDR* (2001), illustrate my point.

- Veterans of Operation Desert Storm, the Vietnam War, the Korean War, and World War II who received no relief from traditional treatment methods found that after EMDR sessions their PTSD symptoms decreased significantly (for a case example, see Part II; Blore, 1997b; Carlson, Chemtob, Rusnak, & Hedlund, 1996; Carlson et al., 1998; Daniels,

Lipke, Richardson, & Silver, 1992; Lipke, 2000; Lipke & Botkin, 1992; Silver, Brooks, & Obenchain, 1995; Thomas & Gafner, 1993; White, 1998; Young, 1995).

- Victims of sexual assault felt relief and were able to resume their lives on all levels (for a case example, see Part II; Edmond, Rubin, & Wambach, 1999; Hyer, 1995; Ironson, Freund, Strauss, & Williams, 2002; Parnell, 1999; Puk, 1991; Rothbaum, 1997; Scheck, Schaeffer, & Gillette, 1998; Shapiro, 1989b, 1991, 1994; Wolpe & Abrams, 1991).

- Surgery patients and accident and burn victims found that once they physically healed, after EMDR they could fully re engage in their lives (Blore, 1997a; McCann, 1992; Puk, 1992; Solomon & Kaufman, 1994).

- Victims of crimes and first responders were able to resolve trauma from assaults (Baker & McBride, 1991; Kleinknecht & Morgan, 1992; McNally & Solomon, 1999; Page & Crino, 1993; Shapiro & Solomon, 1995).

- Children suffering from abuse, assaults, and natural disasters have benefited from EMDR (for case examples, see Chapter 5; Chemtob, Nakashima, & Carlson, 2002; Cocco & Sharpe, 1993; Datta & Wallace, 1994, 1996; Greenwald, 1994, 1998, 1999; Johnson, 1998; Lovett, 1999; Pellicer, 1993; Puffer, Greenwald, & Elrod, 1998; Shapiro, 1991; Tinker & Wilson, 1999; Wilson et al., 2000).

- Mourners struggling with unresolved grief have found that EMDR helped them move on (for a case example, see Part II; Puk, 1991; Solomon, 1994, 1995, 1998; Solomon & Kaufman, 1994; Shapiro & Solomon, 1995).

- Chemical dependents and pathological gamblers have found that EMDR helped them stabilize and reduced their inclination to relapse (Henry, 1996; Shapiro, Volgemann-Sine, & Sine, 1994).

- Artists, athletes, and businesspeople have found that EMDR reduced performance anxiety and enhanced perfor-

mance (for a case example, see Part II; Crabbe, 1996; Foster
& Lendl, 1995, 1996, in press; Maxfield & Melnyk, 2000).

- Phobias: While there is currently little research to substan-
tiate the effectiveness of EMDR with phobias, there is considerable anecdotal evidence that it can be helpful (for a
case example, see Part II).

Only a qualified doctor or therapist can give you the diagnosis of PTSD. But take a look at the following list of questions
and see if any of the following apply to you. If you answer
"yes" to a majority of these questions, you might want to talk
to a professional and seek some guidance and possibly some
EMDR therapy. Sometimes these symptoms can be an indication that trauma has occurred in your life even if you feel that
you haven't experienced anything traumatic. Remember that
trauma is any event that is perceived and held in the body-
mind with symptoms that can disrupt your life.

Checklist of Possible PTSD Symptoms

- I experienced something traumatic that felt life threatening to me. _____
- I witnessed something traumatic that felt life threatening to me. _____
- I see images or memories that feel painful to me. _____
- I have recurring thoughts that seem to take me over so
that I can't focus on what I need to focus on, or the
thoughts repeat over and over and I can't make them
stop. _____
- I feel like the incident is happening to me over and over
in the present. _____
- I find that certain things remind me of the incident and
it upsets me. _____
- Sometimes I feel myself sweat, shake, or have difficulty
breathing when I think of the incident. _____

- I spend time avoiding anything that could possibly remind me of the incident. _____
- I try to not talk about the incident because it is too difficult to talk about. _____
- I feel like I don't enjoy anything in my life anymore. _____
- It's hard to feel close to my family or friends. I tend to feel all alone most of the time. _____
- I find it difficult to feel my feelings, and everything feels flat. _____
- Sometimes I feel like my life will end soon. _____
- I have trouble falling asleep or staying asleep. _____
- I tend to get irritated easily and burst out in anger easily. _____
- I find it hard to concentrate on whatever I'm doing. _____
- I get easily distracted. _____
- I feel like I'm on edge. _____
- I can't relax. I must stay alert at all times. _____
- I am easily startled. _____
- I have nightmares. _____
- I have trouble recalling different aspects of the incident. _____
- I find little joy in the things I do. _____
- I feel as if I have a limited future, like I won't have a career, marriage, or children. _____

CHAPTER THREE

The Phases of EMDR Therapy

We do not believe in ourselves until someone reveals that deep inside us something is valuable, worth listening to, worthy of our trust, sacred to our touch. Once we believe in ourselves we can risk curiosity, spontaneous delight or any experience that reveals the human spirit.

e.e. cummings

In this chapter, I will break down the 8 phases of EMDR so you can become familiar with the steps involved in the therapy. Then I will walk you through a case example of Todd, a client who had experienced an auto accident and came in for EMDR to heal the aftereffects of his traumatic incident. This example will help illustrate the phases of EMDR therapy so you get a better sense of what a client might expect. Remember, every client is unique in his process, so this example is designed to give you a sense of the work and may not exactly represent what your therapy will look and feel like.

Laying the Groundwork

Therapy begins when you enter a therapist's office. Your therapist will want to get to know you so she can help you the best she can. Let's take a closer look at the 2 phases of laying the groundwork, during which your therapist is learning more about you and helping you establish a solid foundation to do safe trauma work. The first is phase 1, client history and then phase 2, preparation.

Phase 1: Client History

With EMDR, there are stages to the healing process. In the beginning, your therapist will ask you personal questions. These questions may seem nosy, but it's important that your therapist know your history. In order to understand and help you, she needs to know what you've experienced in your life that's contributing to how you're feeling and the problems you're struggling with, and to assess your readiness for EMDR. Such questions may include the following:

Current Problem

- Why have you come in for therapy?
- When did your problem begin?
- What was the initial event?
- What are your symptoms?
- When did your symptoms start?
- Is there anything that activates or upsets you currently?
- What are your goals in therapy?

Family History

- What was it like growing up in your family?
- What were your parents like?
- Any significant events that made a lasting impression on you?
- Any history of parents' substance abuse, sexual abuse, or traumas?
- Do you have any history of substance abuse, sexual abuse, or traumas?

Health

- Are you taking any medications presently or have you in the past? If so, which ones?
- Do you have any illnesses?
- What is your self-care regimen?
- Have you ever experienced any accidents or head injuries?

Strengths

- What are the positive memories you have?
- How have you successfully coped with your issues and challenges?
- What do you like about yourself?
- Are there any times you can remember when you felt safe, strong, and competent?
- Do you have any mentors, role models, or people you feel care or cared about you?

Goals

- What do you hope to gain in EMDR therapy?
- How will you know when this therapy is complete?

Therapists will have different ways of getting to know you, and their questions may vary. These questions are just a sample of what your therapist might ask. The history-taking process can take one session or several sessions depending on your unique history and life experiences. These questions are important. Your therapist needs to get to know you and, in addition, the two of you begin to build trust and rapport by sharing this information while the therapist responds with empathy. It has been found that the relationship between therapist and client is key to the foundation of successful therapy. You should feel comfortable with your therapist so that you can begin to trust the therapy and do the work you need to do. When there is a severe trauma history, trust is difficult and may take some time. Most important, you need to feel safe enough to do the EMDR therapy, and your therapist will work with you to create a safe place to do your work. During trauma work you will need to be able to let your therapist know what you are experiencing at any given moment so she can make good decisions about keeping you safe. Through the entire question-and-answer process, if you have any fears and concerns about your treatment you can tell your therapist. Your fears are important and your therapist will want to help support you and make you feel as safe and comfortable as possible.

As I get to know my clients, I begin to see how past experiences have impacted their lives and what they are experiencing today. I want to understand them as best I can. From their answers I can then begin to form a treatment plan. From there the pacing of the treatment is assessed by the needs of the client. Some clients come in for therapy once a week, while others need more and will come in twice a week. Consistency is important when you first start therapy to help build a relationship, trust, and rapport. During this time I also begin to explain EMDR and what the client can expect. Questions from clients are important and I spend as much time as is needed to help them understand the process they are about to undertake.

I let clients know that when something happens that they find disturbing or threatening, like other animals they are genetically programmed to do one of three things: fight, flee, or freeze. It's important to remember that for an event to register in the brain as traumatic, it doesn't have to be a big-T trauma such as combat or an accident. Many day-to-day events can register in the body-mind as little-t traumas, when something happened to you and you were unable to process it for whatever reason. No doubt you've heard it said that beauty lies in the eye of the beholder. Well, trauma lies in the eye of your nervous system. What may feel traumatic to one person may feel like nothing to another, and vice versa. You probably know people who have walked away from accidents and experienced no aftereffects. And then there are people like me who experience a simple event of being stopped by a police officer as traumatic. The important point I make to my clients is this: don't judge yourself or allow other people to convince you that you shouldn't feel the way you feel. If an event feels traumatic or disturbing to you, then it is.

Clients ask me all the time why they just can't get past something. Why does this hurt so much? The answer is this: As best we know now, a disturbing event becomes traumatic when a person's nervous system fails to process some or all of the sensory information—what you saw, heard, smelled, tasted, or felt, as well as your emotions and your thoughts—for whatever reason and it remains locked in your body-mind. Sometimes such information can combine with other remembered information in your brain that may be real or imagined, thereby intensifying the aftereffects of the trauma.

As stated earlier, memory is held in the brain as a web of associations. Let's look at a car crash incident as an example. When someone experiences a car accident, the present experience will be sorted in the brain to see if anything in the past is similar to this event. The past information could be real or imagined. If there is any connection, this memory will join the web of any past memories through association in the "car crash web." Or it might not. That is the mystery of the brain. We can't know for certain until we begin the treatment. The point to remember is that ordinarily your nervous system efficiently and effectively processes your experiences, partly during waking hours as you talk and think things through with other people and partly at night during the REM phase of sleep when dreaming takes place. But sometimes a disturbing experience isn't processed, either because circumstances prevent it or because it's so disturbing that the mind blocks it out. To use an extreme example (because it's so clear and because it was one of the first traumas treated with EMDR), consider combat.

A soldier sees his best friend shot and killed. He's in a war zone and can't sleep for several nights. Also, the death of his friend is so disturbing that he puts it out of his mind. Of course, exactly the opposite has happened. The disturbing event—combat, the death of his friend—has not been put out of his mind, but frozen, locked into his mind and felt through his body as disturbing fragments of memory. Immediately or as time goes by he begins to experience a variety of symptoms that seem to make no sense but interfere with his life. Even though rationally he knows he's safe, he finds himself fearful, unable to sleep, startled by noise, afraid for his family, experiencing nightmares and flashbacks, and feeling guilty and depressed. All these symptoms are past-trauma related and can feel like a trauma is being reexperienced. For this soldier, it can feel as if combat and the death of his friend are happening in the present.

Once a client understands more about trauma and its impact on the body-mind, we can then find targets, which is a term used in EMDR therapy. Targets are identified disturbing events, memories, or issues that have been locked in the memory networks and are disrupting the client's present life. While therapists may approach the identification of targets in different ways, the goal is always the same: to identify the level of disturbance associated with each distressing event, memory, or issue and then choose the order of targets that will offer the greatest and quickest relief of the present symptoms. A treatment plan is discussed from the list of potential targets to be worked on at later dates.

Also during this phase, I start assessing my clients' readiness for EMDR. I evaluate when my clients will be ready to start the desensitization phase by supporting and helping them build the strengths needed to do the reprocessing in EMDR. We identify the issues, memories, and symptoms to be worked on through EMDR so that a treatment plan can be made. I listen to my clients to see what they feel is important to work on while I'm assessing what I think will be helpful to them. Therapy is a collaborative process.

Phase 2: Preparation

As I'm getting to know you as a client, I begin to prepare you for EMDR treatment with skill building. This is a part of the preparation phase and is key to any good trauma therapy. I look at your external and internal strengths, which therapists may call external and internal resources.

Let's look at the external resources first. I want to know how your day-to-day functioning is going and if your basic needs are being met. Having things and people around you that make you feel stable, safe, and secure helps support you to do healing work. Do you have a roof over your head, a stable job, a support team of good friends and family, or are you isolated and struggling to put food on the table? I have found that if these basic needs are taken care of, it's easier to do trauma work. If you are going through a major move or change, it may be too stressful to be trying to heal past wounds when right now all you can think about is how to get your belongings moved. If you are overwhelmed right now, EMDR may not be appropriate, and your therapist can work with you as you stabilize your life. EMDR may be an option after you get settled and develop more support and resources. If your basic needs aren't being met, your therapist may spend time supporting you to make good choices to get resources in place. This may involve practical steps such as getting a job, finding child care, or meeting supportive caring people.

Now let's look at internal resources. Internal resources include your ability to feel strong inside yourself and feel pleasure, joy, and happiness. Sometimes trauma hurts people's ability to feel good or positive about their world or themselves. Negative or painful emotional states become habitual and, for some people, all they know. It is your therapist's job to help you know that it is okay and safe to feel good about yourself. Being able to change emotional states from one feeling to another is an important skill to have. At the end of a long hard day when you feel stressed from work, do you have the ability to come home and find ways to feel better, like putting on your favorite music, making a good meal, talking to a friend, or reading a good book? Are you able to find ways to feel nurtured, safe, and comforted? You might need some help in developing these skills, and the amount of time spent on them depends on your individual needs.

If needed, you will learn to self-soothe, manage your symptoms, be more skilled at self-control, and be able to handle difficult situations more easily and confidently. There are practical steps to help you feel better right away. The amount of resource building will depend on your current situation. The goal is for you to function the best you can in your life and be well prepared for EMDR and the deeper healing that results. Some clients may need very little of this preparation work before moving straight into doing EMDR desensitization, while others may need many sessions to work on strengthening, resources, and just good solid supportive therapy. For example, they might need to do some problem solving, or learn to recognize when they are getting activated, how to set better boundaries, how to communicate more effectively, or how to handle emotions better. Your therapist will help you determine what skills you need and help you explore and develop them in your sessions.

When building internal resources, your therapist will incorporate something called resource development installation (RDI), a procedure that helps a client strengthen any positive internal state by using bilateral stimulation (BLS) to enhance the feeling. Your therapist will guide you to build a strong image or mental picture that represents what you want to be feeling. This image may include whatever sensory information you can identify: colors, sounds, textures, or temperatures. She will then guide you to notice whatever comes into your awareness in that moment. Because I'm a body-centered psychotherapist, I instruct clients to bring this awareness into their body consciousness and allow their posture to reflect how they are feeling. I sometimes have clients experiment with movement to support the felt sense of this awareness. Then I encourage clients to find a word or phrase that reminds them of this experience. It is helpful to have body-mind associations with a word relating to the image, emotions, and posturing. A word or phrase will help you to easily recall this felt sense and return to this feeling. Once you have connected to the image and feel your feelings connected with the resource, your therapist will add BLS to enhance the experience. I like to say, "Let the feeling grow as big as it can get." If you are struggling to stay with a positive feeling, the BLS will not be added right away. You will work toward using BLS as you practice having the positive feelings without it.

Let's look more specifically at these internal resources, which I will go over in detail in this chapter. Your EMDR therapist will help you develop something called a safe place and work with containment skills. The other internal resources that I will mention are not essential to EMDR but are important in trauma work from a body-centered perspective. These additional skills may be addressed if your therapist feels they are important to your healing process. They may include relaxation, belly breathing, grounding, or mindfulness practice. I'm also going to walk you through some experiential exercises in this section, so you can try some of these at home if you wish. You may want to make a CD of your voice saying the script so that you can play it back and do the exercise with your own voice leading you. This can be a way to start preparing for EMDR therapy, increase your self-care, or just become familiar with the resources so when your therapist brings them into therapy you can understand their purpose. These resources are not a substitute for trauma therapy and their purpose is to support and strengthen one's inner sense of self.

Safe Place

A safe place is a real or imaginary place that clients create in their mind's eye that, when imagined, produces a sense of calm, peace, and relaxation in the body-mind. I help every client find a safe place before starting EMDR desensitization. You develop this skill so that you can recall this place and change how you are feeling in the moment whenever you want to. This creates a sense of safety in therapy. For those who have experienced trauma, their sense of the world has changed and may not feel very safe. In that case, I have the client find a name that is comforting. Some other names used for safe place may be inner retreat, peaceful place, soulful place, or whatever works best for you. This exercise can help you feel calmer and more in control of how you feel and how you perceive your world. It is important when you create this imaginary place for yourself that it does not connect to your trauma in any way. It should be a pure image that feels good in body, mind, and soul.

Exercise:
Begin by sitting comfortably in a chair. You can have your eyes open or closed while you are doing this exercise. Begin to think of a place, real or imagined, that you wish you could be in where you feel nurtured, safe, and relaxed in your body. It might be an image, a sensation, or a word. What details do you notice? Is there a temperature? Is there a color? Are there other living beings? Are there any objects you would like with you that help you feel secure and safe? What makes this place safe and nurturing? Check in with your body and notice how it feels. Are you letting go of tension and feeling more ease in your body? Take a deep breath and relax. Let your body move however it needs to in order to support this feeling of relaxation. Is there a word or phrase

that could represent how you feel in this place, or is there a name for this place? Say the word or phrase and see if it feels right. If you were to say it later, would you be able to bring up this image and feel this again? Some examples might be: "I am at peace. Everything is okay. I am relaxed," or "beach, mountains, meadow." There is no right or wrong answer to this, only that it makes you feel good inside when you go there in your mind's eye. Take some deep breaths and enjoy this moment. Stay in your peaceful place as long as you like, making sure you are fully enjoying it. When you are ready, gently and slowly begin to bring yourself back into the present moment by opening your eyes and looking around the room. Feel your feet on the ground, take a deep breath, and enjoy ...

If you can't do a safe place because it's hard to visualize or you can't think of a place that feels good, don't worry. Your therapist will work with you in other ways to help you feel okay. If the word *safe* is difficult for you, try substituting other words that may feel more comforting, like ease, relaxing, calm, peaceful, or serene. Bring that quality into your place. You can also bring in a safe object to feel more secure—like imagining an animal, a rock, or maybe a blanket. Or your therapist may have you imagine something that represents a quality you would like to embrace—for example, feeling strong might evoke an image of an oak tree or a mountain. Or you might incorporate positive memories, such as playing an instrument as a child. One of my clients played the piano and he felt good when he remembered playing his instrument. Finding this relaxed, calm state in your body-mind is the purpose of this exercise so that you can learn to calm your nervous system.

Containment

Containment involves developing a mental picture of an imaginary container into which can be placed upsetting issues, emotions, or thoughts so that they will not interfere with your need to manage your daily life. Learning to do this gives you mastery over your emotional states and creates a sense of control and safety. Containment is an important skill you need to learn before you can begin EMDR. Revisiting a trauma, even in the context of therapy, can be disturbing. When EMDR sessions do not fully process, you may be left with some disturbing images, thoughts, feelings, or sensations. Containment is the skill of learning to put whatever is disturbing into an imaginary container, so that you are able to function better in your daily life between sessions with a sense of well-being and accomplishment. Some people learn containment from their families as they grow up. In other families, however, children learn that one upsetting event ruins everything, all day, and maybe all week.

Another word used for this skill is compartmentalizing. While she was on the TV show *Dancing with the Stars*, Marie Osmond's father passed away. She said, "The show must go on," meaning that she put her grief aside while she performed and then allowed herself to feel her grief later, when there was time for her to express it in the appropriate place. Performers learn this very early on. There were many times when I performed professionally that I had to put something on the back burner and find the focus to perform even when I didn't feel like it. Learning this skill allows you to be able to shift emotional states in the moment so you can be more present with what needs to happen. This does not mean that you are stuffing away your feelings, never to be felt again. Rather, you are allowing yourself to feel more in control of your feelings and are finding appropriate ways to express these feelings and deal with them at a later time.

I help clients imagine a strong container that can hold disturbing thoughts, emotions, and issues, a place that they can come back to later and unpack difficult feelings when they're ready to deal with them in our sessions. Some of the containers my clients have used include a bank vault and a combination lock, a treasure chest locked with a chain, computer disks that can be removed from a computer, and the filing cabinet in my office. One client used a Tupperware container, but when she felt it wasn't strong enough she locked it in a closet. Then she was able to contain the disturbance easily. As you can see, the important thing is to create your container in a way that makes sense to you. You know it works when you can relax, take a deep breath, and feel okay inside. If you have trouble imagining a container, then think about how you transition from one thing to the next throughout your day.

I personally struggle with imagining a container, so I take a deep breath and focus on the here and now; where I am in the room, what I see—colors, shapes, objects. I put my focus on what I am about to do and put what I need to contain away through my thoughts and actions. See what works for you. The following is a containment exercise you can try at home. When you contain, never put a part of yourself in the container, only upsetting issues or feelings.

Exercise:
Begin by slowing down and taking a deep breath. You can have your eyes opened or closed while you are doing this exercise. Begin to imagine in your mind's eye a container that can hold anything that is upsetting you in the moment. What is the shape, size, and texture of this container? Is it big enough to hold what is upsetting you? Is it strong enough? Can you seal the container really tight so nothing can get out? Let your imagination find whatever feels right to you. The important thing is to be able to put the upset in the container and be able to breathe and feel relaxation in your body. So now, imagine putting any upset in this container and see how that feels. Are you able to let go of it and breathe, relax, and feel better? If not, maybe you need a different container. Keep trying until you find the right one. Once you have contained whatever needs to be contained, go back to your safe place and enjoy being there.

In therapy, it is possible to learn to put upsetting pieces of your trauma memory in your container to be worked on in your next session. You can store the feelings that are disturbing until you have time and a safe place to process them. This does not mean that you are stuffing away your feelings and going into denial that something bad has happened. You are learning to compartmentalize the issues so that you build the skill to work on them in an appropriate place and time.

Relaxation

People think when they come to therapy that they are just going to talk about their problems. As a body-centered psychotherapist, I think there are some important skills to learn, and one of them is how to relax your body and mind. When relaxing, you are slowing down as you shift your nervous system from fight or flee to rest and digest. Remember, when you experience a traumatic event you go into fight, flee, or freeze mode. When you process the trauma, you come out of this body reaction. When you don't process the trauma, it can get held in the body-mind and create tension, rigidity, and even pain. Learning to relax your body helps you prepare to do trauma work and brings awareness to the body where areas of distress are being held. The following exercise for relaxation has been adapted from Francine Shapiro's book, *EMDR* (2001).

Exercise:
Sit in a comfortable position. You can do this with your eyes open or closed. Imagine a healing color for today, one that makes you feel good inside when you imagine that color. This color can be different on different days depending on how you feel. Imagine this color above your head and begin to let this color stream into the top of your head. As the color moves in, let it erase any tension and tightness that you might be feeling. Let it melt your tension as if the sun were coming in and melting an ice cream cone. Let your eyes soften, your jaws, cheeks, mouth, roof of your mouth, soften and let go as the color bathes and soothes your head, in-

cluding your brain and all the muscles. Let this color move down your neck, releasing any tension you feel, your throat softening with this healing color. Now let it stream through your arms and out through your fingertips. Bring your attention back to your torso and let this beautiful color stream and bathe your organs, your heart, lungs, liver, intestines. Take your time and really let each organ relax with this energy. Next let the color move down your back and spine releasing any held tension, melting the muscles until they are soft and supple. Give in to the experience and keep letting go as your body fills up with this wonderful color. Now let the color move through your pelvis, legs and down through your feet. The color is now streaming down into earth. Ask your body, is there anything you want to let go of right now in this moment? And then send it down your legs and feet and down into the earth, releasing it and giving it away. You can repeat this several times until you feel completely finished and all you feel is ease in your body and mind. Gently and slowly bring your awareness back into the room, making sure you feel solid in your body as you look around the room.

As you can see, this kind of relaxation is not about relaxing in front of the television. Rather, I am suggesting that you consciously bring your awareness inside to your internal experience and release tension within the body. Sometimes people hold their bodies very tight. This is unconscious and they are shocked when they let themselves feel the difference of letting go. The benefits of relaxation are that you decrease your heart rate, respiratory rate, blood pressure, muscle tension, thinking, and increase alpha wave activity in the brain. Regular practice for 20 minutes a day can help heal your body-mind and make your healing journey more successful.

Belly Breathing

Belly breathing is a wonderful skill that encourages healing. Clients are surprised when I teach them how to change their breathing, because breathing happens unconsciously every day. But when we focus our attention on our breathing and become conscious of it, we can actually change what is happening in our nervous system. Your breathing is the bridge between the unconscious and conscious. When you are afraid, the sympathetic nervous system becomes activated—flight, flee, or freeze—and your breathing will become shallow and more rapid and occur high in your chest. Anxiety and the feeling of fear increase with this type of breathing.

When you breathe in a relaxed way, more fully, from your abdomen, you feel a greater sense of relaxation. This kind of breathing stimulates the parasympathetic nervous system—the branch of the autonomic nervous system that is designed for relaxation and digestion. You will discover that as your breathing deepens, your body begins to relax more and more. You will be able to handle stronger emotional states and stay grounded in your body. You will learn to consciously shift from your sympathetic nervous system to your parasympathetic nervous system—rest and digest.

Exercise:
Sit in a comfortable position. Bring your awareness inside and notice the tension in your body. Put your hand on your abdomen. Begin to notice your breath come in and out of your nose or mouth. Inhale slowly, filling up your lungs, feeling them fill to the bottom—your hand will rise with your belly when this happens. Pause for a moment and then exhale slowly through your nose or mouth. Exhale fully, letting go completely. Do this 10 times in and out. Make it smooth and regular—you can count if this helps you to keep it smooth. Inhale for 3 counts, hold for 3 counts, exhale for 3 counts, and so on. You can increase the length of the inhale and exhale as you master this exercise. If you get lightheaded, stop for a little while, regroup, and try it again. This can take practice. You may not be used to taking in this much oxygen.

I have clients notice their breathing patterns at home to see how shallowly or deeply they are breathing at different moments in the day. Through this awareness, they can begin to feel when their sympathetic nervous system is activated and learn to shift into their parasympathetic nervous system by changing their breathing, which supports their emotional state.

Grounding

Grounding is important to experience because it is the connection you feel to the earth and your own body. As your day progresses, it's easy to lose connection through your legs and feet to the ground. We're busy thinking and doing and our energy rises into our upper body. When you experience trauma, energy goes into different parts of your body. Fight—energy goes to your arms and hands; flee—to your legs and feet; freeze—energy freezes. There are times when an individual will just check out of an experience. This can happen when you feel overwhelmed. It is a survival mechanism and an effective way to continue functioning. Checking out may then become a coping mechanism.

By staying connected to your body and feeling a solid connection to the ground, you can handle more emotional states and process trauma more easily. You can stay more aware of your surroundings, feel stronger and rooted, move through space more confidently, and handle more stressful situations. Grounding can be accomplished by feeling your feet on the ground, imagining roots growing into the earth. You can also ground by holding a favorite object that you associate with a time that you felt strong and competent. Maybe you have a smooth beautiful rock that you hold when you feel stressed, and when you hold that rock you always think of a wonderful trip that you took where you found that rock. You can make contact with the floor by stomping your feet or pushing your hands against a wall to feel the push. Next time you take a walk, slow down and put your awareness in your feet and legs. Can you feel the contact with the earth? Take time and notice. Are you so busy rushing that you can't feel anything? Slow down and feel.

Exercise:
Take a moment to take your shoes off and feel your feet on the
ground. Imagine that you have roots growing from your feet into
the earth. These roots are strong and connect you so that you feel
strong and supported. Let this feeling move up through your
body, making sure you feel strong and connected to the floor.
Slow down and pay attention to this connection. Feel it from your
feet and legs to your torso, feeling the full support of your body.
Slowly walk and feel how your weight shifts from one foot to the
other. Feel how solid you feel, strong, rooted, connected. Look
around and see what you notice when you slow down to feel
grounded. Take this feeling with you wherever you go.

There is a myth in our culture that faster is better. The problem with this concept is that people get ungrounded, make
mistakes, and feel stressed and overwhelmed. When I invite
clients to slow down, though it feels like they won't get everything done, they actually get more done because they use less
energy to do the same task and they become more efficient.
In addition, taking the time to learn how to ground your energy in your body can make trauma work easier and safer.

Mindfulness

There are many types of meditation, and I encourage you to
explore what might feel right for you so that you can develop
the skill of mindfulness. The practice involves slowing down
and bringing awareness internally and becoming more present
in the moment with what is really happening inside of you.
We tend to be focused on worrying about the future or get
stuck in the past with our mind. Learning mindfulness, you
begin to observe your experience and not judge it—just observe it. Experts are finding now that this kind of practice can
be very effective for pain and stress reduction. When you are
traumatized, it can be hard to be mindful. What you feel is the

past trauma taking over, and this makes it hard to stay present. It takes practice to learn to be with yourself, calm your mind, and observe what you are noticing. You will begin to develop an internal witness or observer to your experience. Try the next exercise and notice how you feel in the beginning and how you feel at the end. Many people experience a sense of calm and relaxation while others gain a deeper awareness of their body and mind that they did not have before.

Exercise:
Begin with your eyes open or closed and allow your awareness to move inside your body. Notice the sensation of your seat on the couch. Bring your awareness to your breath as it comes in and out of your nose or mouth. Breathe slowly and deeply allowing your belly to relax. Bring your focus to the top of your head, skull, face, jaw, eyes . . . continue with your neck, shoulders, arms, back, abdomen, thighs, calves, feet . . . just noticing whatever is there. You might feel some tension, pain, heat, tingling, numbness, cold sensations. Just track what you're noticing, and you don't have to change anything, just notice. . . . Spend as much time as you need in each area to get to know what it has to say. When you have tracked inside from head to toe, just sit and take a deep breath. Ask yourself what is the felt sense of your body right now. Be with that feeling. Notice any thoughts that arise. Then bring your attention back to your body and your felt sense. And when you are done, gently and slowly open your eyes and come back into the room to reorient to your present location.

By looking at your external and internal strengths, your therapist will assess when you are ready to proceed to the next phase, assessment. If you are stable in your life, can find a safe place image easily, contain without difficulty, feel your feelings, and stay grounded, you will proceed with EMDR pretty quickly. If you struggle with any of these things, your therapist may spend more time helping you develop these skills to make EMDR easier and more successful for you.

EMDR Trauma Sessions

Now let's take a look at the remaining 6 phases that are part of the EMDR Trauma Sessions: assessment, desensitization, installation, body scan, closure, and re-evaluation. During these phases your therapist will guide you through reprocessing chosen "targets" to completion. Afterwards, each target will be carefully reevaluated to check all work and ensure that the healing is fully integrated.

Phase 3: Assessment

In the assessment phase, the therapist helps the client identify the components of the target. Let's look more closely at the components and the questions a therapist will ask to assess, or what I call set up, the target that will be processed through EMDR.

Your therapist begins by helping you find an image of the traumatic event, memory, or issue and then helps you hone in on that image to find the worst part. I know it's hard to imagine going to the worst part because the tendency is not to want to go to the image at all. But this step is important to begin activating the neural network that is holding that memory so that you can process it with EMDR. When you connect to the image, look around and notice what you see. You might notice colors, textures, temperatures, other people, where you are, your age, or an action or behavior. The image can become richer by gathering any sensory information you can notice to help light up or activate the memory network.

Next your therapist will help you find out what negative belief is associated with the image. A negative belief is a belief you hold about yourself that is not true but feels true and is negative in nature. It is typically an "I" statement, a short statement that can generalize throughout one's life, and is not an emotion. A negative belief feels true in the present moment and brings up disturbing feelings. It is not how others feel about you; rather, it is what you believe about yourself. The negative belief is irrational and not true. These beliefs can hold a lot of power in your life and may feel painful when contacted.

Here is a list of negative beliefs that many clients have thought and reported in EMDR therapy:

- I don't deserve love.
- I am a bad person.
- I am inadequate.
- I am not loveable.
- I am not good enough.
- I am stupid.
- I am a failure.
- I am damaged.
- I deserve bad things.
- I cannot trust myself.

Next your therapist will ask you for a positive belief, or what you would like to believe about yourself once you have moved through the distress of the trauma. Finding a positive belief gives you a sense of direction toward where you want to be in your life and also provides hope that change is possible. A positive belief is about you and is usually an "I" statement. It must be believable and true so that it can be fully integrated into your life. Here is an example of a positive belief that would not work: "I can control everything." That would be impossible, since we can't control everything in our life. A more appropriate positive belief might be, "I make good decisions." When you think of the positive statement, it will bring up positive emotions and can generalize throughout your life.

Here is a list of positive beliefs many clients have worked with in EMDR:

- I am a good person.
- I am worthy.
- I can be trusted.
- I can succeed.
- I now have choices.
- I am strong.
- I did the best I could.
- I can handle it.
- I am okay as I am.
- I am capable.

Your therapist will help you find a positive belief during the setup or assessment of the session. She will then ask you to rate the believability on the Validity of Cognition (VoC) scale. Cognition is a therapy term that means belief. Francine Shapiro developed this scale for EMDR therapy. The measurement scale runs from 1 to 7, where 1 equals false (you do not believe the positive belief) and 7 equals true (you believe the positive belief without any doubt). One goal of EMDR is to reach a VoC of 7 for the positive belief. This scale helps you determine how true the belief feels at the beginning of your session and then at the end of your processing the target. This allows you to know how much change has occurred. Clients' VoC scores tend to be low on the scale in the beginning and higher at the end of sessions. The use of this scale is subjective because there is no right or wrong answer to find. It is just what feels true to you in the moment.

Identifying emotions associated with the image and the negative belief of the traumatic event is the next step. Emotions are different from beliefs. They are feelings. Painful feelings from traumatic experiences tend to be avoided or denied. We push them away in order not to feel them. Recognizing your feelings is important. Can you distinguish between feeling sad, mad, enraged, or frustrated? The following is a sample list of emotions to help you see the difference between beliefs and emotions.

abandoned	affectionate	angry	anxious
betrayed	bored	calm	cautious
courageous	curious	defeated	desperate
discouraged	distressed	ecstatic	enraged
embarrassed	furious	grouchy	guilty
happy	humiliated	hurt	impatient
irate	jealous	joyful	mad
miserable	patient	peaceful	proud
rejected	shamed	shy	sorry
stupid	terrified	tolerant	unappreciated
unhappy	useless	vulnerable	wonderful

Once you name your emotions, your therapist will use another scale to help you discern how disturbing this incident feels to you in the present moment. The scale is called the SUDS scale, or Subjective Units of Discomfort Scale, and was developed by psychiatrist Joseph Wolpe. The scale runs from 0 to 10, with 0 equaling no disturbance and 10 equaling the greatest disturbance. Your therapist uses this scale at the beginning of an EMDR session to help both of you assess how disturbing the components feel in the moment and then during the session only when necessary to gauge how effectively the processing is working. The goal of EMDR is to reduce your SUDS level to as close to zero as possible. Many clients are surprised that a SUDS 10 can go down to a 0. It happens all the time. Again, this scale is subjective in nature and is totally based on your experience. There is no right or wrong answer. Remember, when the train starts in Colorado the SUDS will be high, and when you reach Maine it will be at 0.

The final question while assessing the target asks you to locate the disturbance in your body. For example, you may feel tightness in the jaws, pain in the stomach, constriction in the throat, heat in the chest, or difficulty breathing. Locating the disturbance of the incident in your body helps you become aware of the impact this incident had and where it's being held. This process connects you to the present moment of your experience and helps the processing to be more successful.

Let's take a look at all the questions and the order in which they are asked.

- Finding the worst image: What image represents the worst part of the incident?
- Negative belief: When you think about this image, what words go best with that picture that express your belief about yourself now?
- Positive belief: When you think about this image, what would you like to believe about yourself now?
- Validity of Cognition (VOC) scale: When you think about the incident, how true does that positive belief feel to you now, on a scale of 1 to 7, where 1 is totally false and 7 is completely true?
- Emotions: When you concentrate on the incident and your negative belief, what emotions do you feel now?
- SUDS scale: On a scale of 0 to 10, where 0 equals no disturbance and 10 equals the highest disturbance that you can imagine, how disturbing does it feel to you now?
- Location of body sensation: Where do you feel the disturbance in your body?

As you progress through EMDR, you will become very familiar with these questions. Each time, the questions are asked in a specific order to help you sink into the target traumatic memory in order to activate the neural network in your brain. As you reimagine the image, feel again the associated negative beliefs and emotions, and sense where it is located in your body, you enter ever more completely into the traumatic experience.

There will be times when your therapist will direct you to go back in time to find the earliest time you ever remember having feelings similar to this whole event. Remember, memories can be linked in a web, and the therapist will help you find what I call the root of this issue. A template gets laid down in the memory network and then we act and feel from that template. When there is an earlier target, your therapist will assess this by lighting up the memory network with the image, associated negative belief, emotions, and body sensations. Then you can begin to process the earlier trauma first, clearing the template or root event, and then proceeding to the present issue to be processed. The beauty and power of EMDR is that it accesses the neurology of the brain, even without talking about all of the details of the trauma.

Phase 4: Desensitization

Now that your target is assessed, the processing can begin in the desensitization phase. Your therapist may describe a metaphor to help you understand how the processing happens. In the metaphor I mentioned earlier, you imagine you are on a train and you are looking out the window and letting the scenery go by—the green grass, clouds, streams, and cars. You are just noticing it all. You are safe in the train and you are just watching the scenery go by. The scenery may be an image, thoughts, emotions, or sensations. You are just watching them go by and not fixating on anything in the moment. Some clients like to use the metaphor of a movie shown on a screen. You are watching the scenes of a movie go by. Use whatever works for you. The important thing is that movement of some kind is happening and that you are not fixating on anything in particular. You do not have to make anything happen; rather, trust the process.

EMDR therapists assume that the brain is geared toward resolution and healing, as it is with physical ailments. While no one is yet sure just how this works, this processing of healing certainly seems to be true based on years of EMDR experience. As you let go and follow the process, images, thoughts, emotions, and sensations begin to melt out of their frozen state, presumably as they do when you dream. Your subjective experience as you observe this process may seem like sitting in a train looking out the window at a passing landscape. The BLS moves the train and you observe the passing scenery and memories of the trauma as you observe them. Then they disappear. During this ride, you might experience intense emotions, or see scary images, or remember something unexpected and disturbing, or feel strange body sensations that seem to have no physical cause. If this happens, your therapist will encourage you to continue with the process and allow the experience to unfold. She is there to guide, support, and encourage you as you go through the process of integrating each traumatic memory.

The desensitization occurs through a series of sets. A set represents the time you process images, thoughts, emotions, and physical sensations while receiving BLS. Sets can be short or long and can employ different types of BLS that can be fast or slow, intense or weak, depending on your response and your therapist's judgment. Remember, it can be done with eye movement, the Tac/Audio Scans, or with hand taps. You will have a stop signal so that you can stop the process whenever you want to. Your stop signal may be opening your eyes if your eyes are closed, or raising your hand slightly, or nodding your head; whatever you and your therapist agree upon.

Some clients like to do desensitization with their eyes open, others with their eyes closed. You and your therapist will determine how long the BLS set runs. You will discover together what duration and intensity of BLS sets are most effective. When the BLS stops, it's as if the train you're riding has stopped. Each time you stop, you have completed a BLS set. After each set your therapist will check in with you to gauge how the process is going. I always ask for clear feedback about what a client is noticing now. In EMDR there is no need for you to tell your therapist about the entire train ride you just experienced.

This is a major difference between EMDR and talk therapies.

Talk therapy places a premium on verbal descriptions in order to bring to consciousness all that you experienced. This is not necessary with EMDR. After you complete a set, your EMDR therapist will want to know what you are noticing in the moment. There is no right or wrong answer at this point. The client will mention what is happening, which might include a new image, thought, feeling, or body sensation. Every person processes in her own unique way. For some there may be lots of images, while others may just experience pure body sensations. Nothing is "supposed to" happen in any given set. Therefore, it's very important to tell the truth about your experience so that your therapist can make adjustments as she guides you through the process. The sets will continue through that session (and perhaps other sessions) until the body-mind charge associated with the target is reduced to neutral.

As you take this journey, your therapist is your guide and will support you to follow whatever is happening. In the desensitization there is really nothing for you to do but allow your brain to complete its own process, unwinding the trauma while you're experiencing the BLS. The BLS is working with the neurology of your brain; given bilateral stimulation, your brain knows what to do and will do it. Your only job is to report as accurately as you can what's happening between sets. If images, thoughts, emotions, or sensations begin to overwhelm you, signal this to your therapist to stop. She will guide you so that you will feel safe enough to proceed with the processing. At the end of a session, if anything still feels disturbing, she will ask you to contain the disturbance and relax for a time in your safe place so that the target can be completed at your next session. A few EMDR targets will complete in one session, but some will require several sessions.

How will you know when you've reached a neutral state? Your therapist will use the SUDS scale to assess the intensity of a disturbing target, and then use it again only when needed to help gauge when the processing is completed. The goal of

EMDR is to reduce your SUDS level concerning a traumatic event to as close to zero as possible. You will not forget the past traumatic event, but when you remember it, the memory will no longer retain the power that was so disturbing. You will remember the event from a present-day perspective. While some of the frozen trauma dissipates and is discarded, some will also "melt" into your memory so that you remember what happened and that the symptoms of the trauma will be reduced or disappear.

Phase 5: Installation

If you successfully completed the desensitization by reporting a SUDS zero, you will naturally move into the next phase, called installation. The installation phase of EMDR treatment is designed to complete any processing needed and to increase a client's internal strength by replacing the negative self-beliefs associated with the trauma with positive self-beliefs. How does this happen? You hold a new positive self-belief in your mind's eye (that you found during the assessment phase) at the same time as you think about the original traumatic event or memory, while the therapist applies BLS. If this belief has changed during the desensitization phase, your therapist will inquire about this and help you find the most accurate positive self-belief in this phase to install. Your therapist will check in with you to get a sense of how true the positive self-belief feels using the VoC scale. As I explained before, the scale runs from 1 to 7, where 1 equals false (you do not believe the positive belief) and 7 equals true (you believe the positive belief without any doubt). If EMDR has been successful, the traumatic memory should be sufficiently desensitized so that the positive belief reaches a VoC of 7. This phase addresses past traumatic memories or issues, present triggers, and future fears or situations; when complete, you feel at peace with the past, empowered in the present, and able to make healthy choices in the future.

This is an organic process, and the new positive belief integrates during this phase. Many clients experience this phase as feeling wonderful. Some clients find it difficult to trust this new belief because for a long time the negative self-belief associated with the trauma felt so true. Some clients feel a new sense of empowerment at this point and others may want to check out this new viewpoint and test how it feels in the real world. I have had clients tell me months later that they really understand and feel the difference through having life experiences that support this new belief.

Phase 6: Body Scan

Once you have felt the positive new thoughts and feelings and have strengthened them with the BLS, it is time to finish the target with a body scan. This is only done if the desensitization and installation phases are complete. Your therapist will ask you to bring up the original target event paired with the positive belief and scan through your body as though you are in an X-ray machine to see if you feel any residual tension, distress, or discomfort that didn't get processed fully. You will report this to your therapist. If there is any disturbance left, your therapist will help you find a way to release this distress by using BLS. If any new material related to the incident or completely new information arises, your therapist will make a note of this and ask you to put that information and disturbance in your container to be examined at the next session.

Phase 7: Closure

You are now done with your work for the session, and it is time to leave and move into your life again. You will have time to debrief the work you just did and assess how you are feeling. I check to make sure clients feel solid and can move on with their day. I explain that the processing will continue and I encourage them to notice anything that comes up through dreams, thoughts, memories, or whatever comes to mind. I instruct clients to make a note of anything that arises in connection to the work and bring it next time. If the session completed to full installation of the positive belief, I ask clients to be aware of this new belief and how they feel in their everyday life. This might be in relationship to work, home, or play. The therapist encourages the client to support this new feeling in both body and mind.

In some EMDR sessions, the processing (desensitization and installation) is not complete and full resolution is not attained. Your SUDS score will be higher than a zero or one. If that happens, there is no reason for concern. Your therapist will end your session by instructing you to place the disturbance and any unresolved images, thoughts, feelings, and sensations in your container, and then to go to your safe place. Containment prevents you from remaining open and vulnerable to disturbing feelings, and returning to your safe place helps you feel safe during the week before your next session.

I like to check in with clients to see what they are going to be doing after our session, what problems could arise, and how they will take care of themselves. I ask them to jot down anything that arises during the week that seems connected to our work for further processing. If after any session you continue to feel disturbed and overwhelmed, call your therapist so that she can help you contain better and make sure you have another appointment scheduled to resolve what needs to be completed.

Some clients feel refreshed and energized after a session, but others feel tired and want to rest. Remember, EMDR is a neurological process and the effects may continue after a session. You might dream, or new insights might come to you. Other memories might rise into consciousness. If any of these do occur, just jot them down and bring them to your next session. You and your therapist can decide if any of them hold a charge sufficiently disturbing to necessitate EMDR. Remember that taking time after your sessions to allow your body-mind to integrate what you just processed is important. You may feel a little tender or more vulnerable than usual, so you will want to take care of yourself after your therapy session. Don't rush back to work or make a big decision. Take a walk, have a nice meal, meditate, or do whatever feels good to you. You need time for you. Let this journey have the space it needs so you get the most benefit from your EMDR therapy.

Phase 8: Reevaluation

The final stage of EMDR is reevaluation. When you come in for your next session, your therapist is going to check in with you and ask you what you noticed after your last session. Your therapist will recheck the work you did last week to make sure it is completed, or you may continue to finish an incomplete session from the last time. Your therapist will want to know if any dreams occurred, or if any new memories, thoughts, or insights arose. What successes, new feelings, or thoughts have you noticed? It is important for you to notice whether you are feeling change and what is changing. You may need time to process the last session with your therapist, talking about what you have noticed, or you may be ready to dive in and do more work. This pacing will be determined as you go along.

The Process of EMDR Therapy: Todd's Car Accident

Now that I've taken you through the phases and steps of EMDR therapy, let's look at Todd's story to illustrate what the EMDR therapy phases and process actually looked like for him.

Laying the Groundwork

Phase 1: Client History

Todd, 40 and single, came to see me because he'd been in a car accident 5 years ago. Since then, he had been struggling with anxiety each time he had to drive. After working with him over time, his massage therapist realized that he was still badly traumatized and suggested that EMDR might help. Although he was unfamiliar with the therapy, he decided it was worth a try.

Because Todd knew the source of his trauma, I asked him to tell me the story of his accident as a part of getting to know him. He told me that he'd been coming home from a camping trip and was speeding along a two-lane country road in southern Colorado. The camp had been a spiritual retreat. He remembered as he drove that what he really wanted to do was process and write notes about what had transpired. He said that he felt "not very grounded" and recalled that his attention was "all over the place." Fortunately, he was the only one on that stretch of lonely road. But suddenly a yellow bird appeared in his lane. He couldn't bear to hit it, so he swerved into the opposite lane. But the bird flew in front of him again and this time when he swerved back, the car fishtailed and he lost control. He took his foot off the gas but didn't hit the brake because he was afraid he would roll over. Going 65 miles an hour, swinging wildly back and forth, he kept expecting the car to slow but it never did. He wasn't sure if he was going to live or die in that moment. Finally, he missed a curve and slammed into a ditch.

He felt disoriented but then discovered that he was sitting upright in his car facing back the way he had come. The engine had stalled but the radio was still playing. He realized that the soil was soft from recent rain; it was this earth cushion that had reduced the force of the impact and kept the car from rolling. But the mud under his tires prevented him from driving the car out of the ditch. As he sat there waiting for rescue, he felt amazed to still be alive and relieved that he wasn't physically hurt.

Todd borrowed a friend's car while his car was being repaired. Almost immediately he realized that every bump in the road startled him and that the more he drove, the tenser he became. He went to a massage therapist to deal with his muscular tension. As time went on, however, his anxiety began to border on fear and his emotional and physical responses started to get the best of him. Quite rational, he kept telling himself that he was okay, and he knew that that was the truth. The trouble was, his body-mind did not agree. Every time he got into a car, he responded as if something terrible was about to happen. His heart raced; he broke into a sweat; he gripped the steering wheel and found himself holding his breath until he could get out of the car. Clearly, Todd was experiencing a trauma response. His body was reacting to every common driving experience as if it was the car accident all over again.

I delved into his personal and medical history to make sure he didn't have a head injury. In addition to many other questions, I asked if he'd had any other accidents or traumas. Very often a traumatic event like this can reactivate similar traumas from the past. That wasn't the case here. Todd had no history that would connect to this current trauma as far as I could tell. Todd's trauma—the automobile accident—had been a single traumatic incident. Barring the unforeseen, the treatment would probably move relatively quickly and easily.

It was clear that Todd could not literally fight or flee from his car when it was out of control. He clearly was unable to escape and became frozen, fearing for his life. This was clearly a disturbing event. But he wanted to know why he couldn't "just get past it" and have things back to normal. I explained what happens when a traumatic event occurs and how he did what he could to survive. I told Todd that for some reason his nervous system was unable to process the car crash experience. Sensory information froze in his nervous system and his body-mind began to respond, first with muscle tension and then with anxiety that soon made it all but impossible for him to drive.

Todd had a stable life. He had a steady job, a good relationship, and a great circle of friends. He felt confident about himself, except that he was struggling with this accident. He didn't have any previous history that I could learn from our talking that could be linked to this event. After I heard Todd's story, I helped him understand what was happening, assured him that EMDR might be helpful, and predicted that if he would trust the therapeutic process he could soon count on driving as he had before the accident. Todd and I felt comfortable that he was ready to do this work.

Phase 2: Preparation

To prepare Todd for EMDR therapy, we began with finding his safe place. At first he thought the notion was hokey and saw no need for it. But as we talked, he remembered a place he loved, where he felt safe: in the woods sitting on a log by a stream listening to the sounds of the water, feeling the breeze, and watching the animals. As he sank into this image, he said it felt really good and he began to enjoy it. We added bilateral stimulation. He liked the pulsers, strengthening his experience of this peaceful place. As he felt the stimulation, he got in touch with the feeling even more strongly and enjoyed it more fully. As it happened, Todd enjoyed his safe place so much and became so skilled at evoking it that he began to use it when something upset him during the week.

Next we added a container for Todd. He chose an imaginary large box that he could close and lock. Whenever something bothered him, he'd just say, "box it up" and it was contained. The more he practiced, the more he appreciated what this skill also had to offer him in his daily life.

That Todd was able to use his safe place and container on his own demonstrated to me that he was ready to move forward in the treatment process. Because Todd knew how to meditate and included massage therapy in his self-care regimen, I knew he could relax his body and that I didn't need to spend time teaching him these skills. I felt confident that Todd had ample inner and outer strength and enough resources that we could begin to work on helping him move through his trauma.

EMDR Trauma Session

Phase 3: Assessment

Now that I'd gathered Todd's history and he'd learned to go to his safe place and contain disturbing thoughts, feelings, and issues, we were ready to work with the identified targets. We knew Todd's primary target was the accident. We first decided on a stop signal that he could use if he felt overwhelmed or needed to check in with me—as the client you will always be in control and able to stop the session whenever you feel the need. Todd told me that he would close his eyes during the BLS and open them only if he needed to stop. For BLS, he preferred the Tac/Audio Scan pulsers rather than eye movement or tapping. We now were ready to begin the assessment and desensitization phase of the work. I asked him questions so that he could access the feelings of the experience and light up the memory network so we could desensitize it:

- Finding the worst image: What image represents the worst part of the incident? "My hands glued to the steering wheel and I know something bad is going to happen."
- Negative belief: When you think about this image, what words go best with that picture, words that express your negative belief about yourself now? "I'm stupid."
- Positive belief: When you think about this image, what positive thing would you like to believe about yourself now? "I'm alive and I'm okay."
- VoC scale: When you think about the incident and repeat your positive belief, on a scale of 1 to 7, where 1 is totally false and 7 is completely true, how true do those words ("I'm alive and I'm okay") feel to you now? "3."
- Emotions: When you concentrate on the image—your hands glued to the steering wheel knowing something bad

is going to happen—and your negative belief—"I'm stupid"—what emotions do you feel now? "Fear!"

- SUDS scale: On a scale of 0 to 10, where 0 equals no disturbance and 10 equals the highest disturbance that you can
imagine, how disturbing does it feel now? "10."
- Location of body sensation: Where do you feel the disturbance in your body? "I feel frozen all over. My heart's
racing."

Phase 4: Desensitization

After we assessed the target, I asked Todd to connect to the
image, the words "I'm stupid," and the sensations he was feeling in his body. He started connecting more and more deeply
to the memory of the accident. I asked him to tell me when he
was ready to begin the desensitization and he nodded his head
that he was ready. At this point, I turned on the pulsers to
begin the BLS.

As the set proceeded, I watched as he entered into his traumatic experience. Words were unnecessary. As a body-centered
psychotherapist, and like other EMDR therapists, I have learned
to perceive subtle shifts that occur throughout the body. As
Todd's set continued and emotional waves moved through his
body, I tracked what was happening in order to make sure he
stayed present with his experience and felt safe. Todd was
quiet but I could see that he was processing the traumatic
event. His arms twitched ever so slightly. His eyes were
squeezed shut, his jaw and hands clenched, and his breathing
rapid and shallow. During this initial phase, some clients need
very short sets of BLS, around 30–45 seconds, while others
need more extended sets that can last much longer. There is
no right or wrong timing of the set length. The body-mind
knows what it's doing and I'm trained to help a client like
Todd work with what is right for him.

Todd's first set of BLS lasted a couple of minutes. Although
he was very quiet, through subtle shifts in his body I could

see that he was having an internal experience. I stopped the BLS and asked, "What do you notice now?"

"My fear has increased and my chest hurts."

I told him to go with that; that is, to reenter the body-mind state that he was then experiencing.

The next BLS set lasted longer. I could see the pain in Todd's face. His breath quickened and grew shallow but he continued until his face relaxed and he took a deep breath. I checked in after the set.

"What do you notice now?" I asked.

"I'm going to die and I won't get a chance to say good-bye to anyone."

"Go with that."

Another BLS set lasted a couple of minutes.

"What do you notice now?"

"Somehow I'm alive and I can't make sense of it; I feel confusion; how can this be?"

"Go with that."

I started the BLS. This time the set was very long. As it continued, I noticed slight trembling in Todd's legs and torso that persisted for several minutes. This told me that he was moving through another piece of the trauma. Finally, he stopped and checked in with me.

"What do you notice now?"

"The fear is gone, but I feel tremendous pressure in my head and chest."

"Go with that."

I resumed the BLS. The trembling in his legs continued and his breathing became short and shallow. After a few moments he took a long, deep breath and opened his eyes. I stopped the BLS.

I repeated the same question: "What do you notice now?"

"The pressure has lessened and I feel relief. But I feel stuck with the image in the car."

"Go with that."

As Todd continued with the BLS, tiny shifts occurred in his body. His shoulders lifted toward his ears and then relaxed as his hands clenched the pulsers, and his feet made small running movements. It was as if he was surfing emotions that were being expressed through physical sensations and movements that would only stop when the emotional wave came to an end.

"What do you notice now?"

"I'm angry at myself for being so careless and going too fast; this should have never happened."

Same instruction, another set, and when he stopped, the same question.

"It was just an accident," he said. "It could have happened to anyone. I'm just a little sad."

"Go with that," I told him. After the next set, I asked him, "What do you notice now?" Todd replied, "I feel fine, and I'm okay."

Did he feel fine? Was he okay? With any client who reaches this stage in the healing process, I always suggest, "All right, let's go back to the target." With Todd I said, "When you think of the accident now, is there anything disturbing?"

Todd said, "No, I feel fine. Nothing disturbing." I instructed him to do another set of BLS and just notice if anything else arose. He reported, "nothing."

I then asked him to rate his disturbance on the SUDS scale. "On a scale from 0 to 10 where 0 is no disturbance or neutral and 10 is highly disturbing, how disturbing is this to you now?" His rating was zero. Because this was a single trauma incident, I was not surprised. With no memory networks linked to the event, Todd could move through it from beginning to end without any associated memories surfacing that also would need to be processed. A SUDS rating of zero told me that the desensitization was complete and we could move on to the next phase of the reprocessing, installation.

Phase 5: Installation

Todd had just done a big piece of work and his natural process in the body and mind was moving toward a more adaptive response and a more positive state of being. He started with wanting to believe he was alive and okay.

I asked him, "When you think of the accident and, at the same time, the words 'I'm alive and I'm okay,' are those words still what you want to believe, or is there something better now?" He stated, "That feels right."

I asked Todd, "Okay, when you think about the accident, on a scale from 1 to 7, where 1 equals totally false and 7 equals completely true, how true does "I'm alive and I'm okay" feel now?"

Without hesitation Todd replied, "6." At the start of this session it had been a 3, so this meant that positive change had definitely occurred.

To reinforce this positive belief we did some sets of BLS, and continued until he reported that his positive self-belief had reached a solid 7.

Phase 6: Body Scan

I now had Todd bring up the original incident with the positive belief. When he felt this, I had him turn his attention inward and scan his body for any residual tension or any disturbance that might not have been processed in our work. He mentally scanned his body and stated that he felt fine from head to toe. "No tension." We were done with this piece. It was time to move on to present-day triggers and the future scenarios of the installation phase.

I reminded Todd of the things he had told me that triggered a disturbing response when driving. He had said, "Whenever I drive to work, to friends, to the grocery store, everywhere!" We made a list of each of these present-day triggers and assessed them for processing disturbances he felt while imagining them. We then targeted each one of these triggers until all were fully processed and he felt no disturbance, and with each target we completed an installation. He was able to feel "alive and okay" in each situation. We did further sets of BLS to deepen his body-mind's integration of this positive self-belief. I encouraged him to feel his new sense of confidence in his body and reflect in his posture this new way of being. With each target, a body scan uncovered no new disturbance.

Now he was ready to move into the future. Todd knew that he'd soon be attending another spiritual retreat in the mountains. From his previous experience he anticipated that the road would be bumpy and winding, and as he imagined the drive he began to feel a little anxious. I then had him imagine the journey from beginning to end. I asked him to see in his mind's eye the roads he was going to take, to feel how successfully he would drive them, and then to pair these images and sensations with his positive self-belief of "I'm alive and I'm okay." I had Todd run this "mental video" four times with BLS until he felt secure and confident that he could make the trip without any emotional upset.

All this sounds less dramatic than it was. Like so many other clients, as Todd worked with his positive self-belief he began to feel changes throughout his body-mind. I encouraged this, using BLS to help him feel the new positive self-belief from head to toe, and to integrate all of the changes he had made. This is often when EMDR seems magical to clients. It certainly did to Todd, as he took from EMDR therapy not only relief from symptoms of past trauma, but also a new freedom in the present, as expressed by his positive self-belief: "I'm alive and I'm okay!"

Phase 7: Closure

I reminded Todd that he had done a big piece of work that day and that with EMDR, the processing continues after we are done. I told him to notice his dreams, thoughts, and any new memories to see if anything else came up connected with our work. The next time we would assess this information to see if anything was unfinished that would need to be addressed in a future session. I reminded him that he might feel more sensitive than normal and that he needed to do good self-care that evening. He said he was going home and resting. I also told him that he might feel really energized or really tired and not to be concerned by that, just to notice. He felt eager to leave our session and test our work by driving home and seeing if the EMDR really worked.

Phase 8: Reevaluation

Because Todd's trauma had been a single event without any associated web of memories, he was able to process it in one EMDR session. His anxiety and physical symptoms disappeared completely. After his weekend in the mountains he came in to report that he had driven through stiff winds over dirt roads and felt nothing but confident ease. After months of driving in all sorts of circumstances he continued to feel the same confidence. In fact, he found EMDR so powerful and effective that he decided to continue with therapy to clear some other past disturbing events that still had power and were interfering with his life.

CHAPTER FOUR

Why EMDR Works

*No one saves us but ourselves. No one can and no one may.
We ourselves must walk the path.*

Buddha

After a number of years, most clinicians and
scientists are now convinced that EMDR successfully heals
trauma. But there's a great deal of controversy about why.
How exactly does the EMDR desensitization process—the use
of bilateral stimulation, or BLS, while recalling traumatic memories—actually work? Research is currently underway that may
eventually answer this question, much of it quite sophisticated, using brain scans and other high-tech devices. In the
meantime, a number of theories have been offered to explain
why EMDR is so effective.

Originally, Shapiro developed EMDR using eye movements
as a bilateral form of stimulation. Remember that she recognized that her eyes moving back and forth were helping her
process upsetting thoughts and feelings. Soon, when some
people couldn't coordinate their eyes to move quickly enough,
she had clients follow her fingers. For years EMDR therapists
used only eye movements, but now many use other methods

such as tactile pulsers held in the hands, audible sounds or music, or hand taps on the hands or knees.

Once you have found the BLS method that feels best for you, your therapist will guide you to focus your attention inside. It's like focusing a lens on what is happening inside you in the moment. Through the lens you'll notice pictures, emotions, beliefs, and body sensations. But don't worry if you can't "see inside" in the beginning; your therapist will help you learn how to do this work. As you focus, your therapist will activate the BLS. The process itself is deceptively simple. You focus on an internal state, usually a memory associated with a traumatic event, while your body-mind is simultaneously stimulated with some type of BLS.

You might be working on a positive feeling or working on something more difficult. The funny thing about BLS is that when you focus on the positive aspects they feel like they are growing and expanding, getting stronger and clearer. But when you focus on the disturbing pieces they begin to diminish in power and gradually transform into something new, and you feel empowered.

Over time, EMDR therapists have found no difference in the effectiveness of one BLS method over another. Although only eye movements have been thoroughly studied, therapists and researchers are starting to question if movement of the eyes is truly the key to successful EMDR processing. Uri Bergmann, an independent EMDRIA-approved trainer, has hypothesized that perhaps it's the shifting of attention through bilateral stimulation that jump-starts the brain to begin integrating the trauma, rather than the actual eye movement (Bergmann, 1998). Only more research will clarify this issue, but for now therapists are using different BLS modalities and finding that they get great results.

Now let's take a look at some theories about why EMDR is so successful.

REM Sleep

Researchers are doing animal and human studies to determine if rapid eye movement (REM) sleep can tell us something about why EMDR is effective. REM is a phase of the normal sleep cycle. During REM the eyes flicker from side to side in response to brain activity. It has been postulated that during REM sleep some types of memory are being processed (Maquet et al., 1996). The electrical activity of the brain during REM creates a theta rhythm. This can be observed in the hippocampus (Winson, 1985). It appears that this theta rhythm activates the amygdala area of the brain and that REM sleep is disturbed by traumatic events. When that happens, information that would ordinarily be processed and integrated becomes distorted, first in memory and secondarily by emotional and cognitive interpretations. Because the memory of the actual event is locked in the amygdala, the prefrontal cortex is unable to mediate it; the rational part of your brain shuts down and is not able to help the amygdala sort through the feelings to be processed and integrated.

Researchers used to believe that traumatic memories were permanently locked in the amygdala (LeDoux, 1994). Now, however, they are finding that this is not true. Uri Bergmann postulated that bilateral stimulation creates a state in the brain similar to REM sleep, thereby activating the amygdala and other parts of the brain so that memories previously locked in the amygdala can be freed and begin to integrate (Bergmann, 1998). He believes that by activating the amygdala while guiding a client's attention to the disturbing emotions and body sensations related to a traumatic incident—emotions and sensations that as memories are locked in the body-mind—BLS stimulates the brain to jump-start the process of memory integration, calms the limbic system, and allows the prefrontal cortex to get on with its higher functioning and integrate the memories.

Orienting Response

It has been hypothesized that bilateral stimulation provokes an orienting response, a reflex that brings about an immediate physiological and behavioral response to the slightest change in the environment. It's postulated that repeated presentations of the same stimulus result in a gradual decline in what's termed response magnitude; in the case of trauma, this means the severity of the emotional and physical symptoms when stimulated by unresolved and dis-integrated memories. The idea is that while a person continually remembers and responds to the trauma, BLS stimulation disrupts the orienting response and begins to allow processing to occur (Shapiro, 2001). When the brain perceives that there is no actual current threat, the body-mind will relax. It has also been suggested that the orienting response interrupts past associations to negative thoughts and emotions and permits the development of a new relationship to past stimulation (i.e., memories of the traumatic event), thereby integrating the trauma memories into long-term memory (Barrowcliff, Gray, Freeman, & MacCulloch, 2001). BLS facilitates a response that's more adaptive than trauma symptoms and encourages a fuller understanding and a new meaning for an old situation (Stickgold, 2002).

Stimulation of Both Sides of the Brain

Another hypothesis is that by stimulating both hemispheres of the brain, BLS allows what is stuck to become more agile, thereby freeing the system for integration; that eye movement activates the hippocampus and stimulates the process of memory evaluation and consolidation to realign; and that somehow BLS allows focus on inner emotional states while simultaneously increasing the brain's alertness and ability to metabolize whatever is being remembered (Parnell, 2007).

Finally, it has been proposed by Bruce Perry, an internationally recognized authority on children in crisis, that the very rhythm of the BLS mimics drumming and dancing, which in many cultures is used to help process traumatic memories. The back-and-forth stimulation has a calming effect on the nervous system and can short circuit the trauma response (Parnell, 2007).

The fact remains that more research is necessary and is being done as we speak. What's important to remember, however, is that no matter what the final explanation proves to be, EMDR works. Millions of people have already benefited and so, perhaps, can you.

CHAPTER FIVE

How EMDR Differs From
Other Therapies

Wherever you go, go with all your heart.

Confucius

The most common forms of therapy being
taught in colleges and universities today are psychodynamic
psychotherapy and cognitive behavioral therapy. Both have
strong histories describing how they developed and how they
work.

Psychodynamic psychotherapy evolved from the work of
early pioneers in psychology like Sigmund Freud and Carl
Jung. Although there are many variations, the theory underlying all of them is that any present life dysfunction is rooted in
or linked to the past. It's also assumed that a great deal of
what's important to know in order to make change is unconscious, either because it has been suppressed (consciously forgotten) or repressed (forgotten without conscious awareness).
The principal method of treatment is conversation between
client and therapist; thus the sometimes pejorative term "talk
therapy." But it's the nature of these conversations that's considered important. Together, client and therapist explore the
client's current thoughts, feelings, and behaviors, often focusing on childhood, in order to see how earlier experiences have

influenced who the client is today. To discover unconscious information, the therapist uses techniques such as free association and dream interpretation and permits the client to establish a strong emotional bond with her. This is called transference. The theory is that the client transfers the emotions he felt as a child toward his parents onto the therapist and by so doing can be "reparented" in a more positive way, working through conflicts with the therapist that he could never resolve with his parents. The underlying assumption is that by encouraging the awareness of unconscious material that's causing dysfunction, allowing strong emotions to arise and cathartically release, and employing language, metaphor, and symbolism to make sense of the client's history and current experience, the client will be healed. That is, he will become conscious of what was unconscious and, therefore, free of whatever unconscious conflicts have made his life dysfunctional.

While it was a profound breakthrough in the 19th century, psychoanalysis and all of the psychodynamic therapies that evolved from it through the years have fallen into some disfavor. While talk therapy remains probably the most common form of psychotherapy practiced today, and many have found it quite helpful, it has been criticized for a number of reasons. Four of the most prominent criticisms are these: (1) the therapy's underlying assumption—current dysfunction arises from unresolved (and often unconscious) conflicts in the past—is either untrue or at least impossible to prove or disprove; (2) other than a client reporting that he feels better, there is no way to measure the success of the therapy; (3) the therapy relies heavily on sophisticated conceptual and language skills—understanding symbolism, the use of metaphor—beyond the ability of many clients; and (4) it takes too long and costs too much.

Psychologists dissatisfied with psychodynamic psychotherapy developed cognitive behavioral therapy (CBT), which evolved from earlier rational emotive therapy. CBT blends different techniques to help clients change their irrational, negative, and false thought patterns into thought patterns that are rational, positive, and true. The theory is that as a person's thoughts change, his behaviors will change too. Or, conversely, if a person changes his behaviors, his thoughts will change. The underlying assumption is that problems in living are the result of conditioned responses—that is, a person learns negative and false thoughts and behaviors that he then generalizes, rendering his life more or less dysfunctional. The therapeutic goal of CBT is to help a client learn to manage his emotions by changing his thoughts and behaviors. Although CBT also relies on talk as its primary method, here there is no need for the client to know the (unconscious) cause of his emotions or behaviors. Why you feel or act the way you do is irrelevant. What's important is that you change your thoughts and behavior. If you do that, your life will change for the better.

Research has shown that CBT is an effective treatment choice for relieving PTSD symptoms. Helping people learn to identify their irrational thinking patterns and replacing them with rational ones is an important step in healing trauma.

Body-Centered Psychotherapies

Over the last 20 years, body-centered therapies have become widely accepted as a way to work with trauma. Research on memory and trauma supports the importance of including the body in the therapeutic process. To help deal with unresolved trauma, body-centered therapies consider a client's body postures, movements, gestures and physical sensations to be as important as what he says, if not more so. The theory is that as the client becomes increasingly aware of emotions related to trauma as expressed in physical sensations and emotionally charged images, this deepening awareness in and through the body will allow and encourage the transformation of unresolved emotions and negative beliefs related to a traumatic event. The goal is to release emotions held in the body—

muscles, cells, and joints, wherever the memory of trauma is being held. Then the client will be able to move through the trauma to find resolution through discharging what was held in the body as trauma. By going into the body and trusting that the body will show the way to healing, cognitive awareness will arise naturally through the process so that the whole experience can be integrated. New body posturing and movements will occur as a result, helping clients feel and behave differently. At this point there is little empirical research to support the effectiveness of body-centered work as a trauma treatment. There are, however, many anecdotal case studies to support that body-centered psychotherapies can heal traumatic symptoms. Bessel van der Kolk, world expert in the field of trauma, is supporting some body-centered therapies as important approaches to healing trauma.

EMDR as an Integrative Therapy

In EMDR, I believe that Francine Shapiro has integrated aspects of talk and body therapies into a method that values the body-mind connection. EMDR has retained the best of psychodynamic and CBT therapies and psychological education to help clients think more effectively. The paradox is that while variations of talk therapy form the basis of EMDR, during the desensitization phase the client needs to talk very little. An important therapeutic benefit of EMDR is that if you prefer, or find it too stressful, you don't have to relive your trauma by telling your therapist every detail of the traumatic event. Trauma can be processed privately, internally, and still be healed. As an EMDR client, your chief task is to monitor your inner body-mind experience. Talk need only be used to communicate what is happening during your check-in so that your therapist can guide you through the process. It's an EMDR therapist's job to help you track your trauma responses while at the same time creating a safe environment so that you will move through the trauma. This includes trauma symptoms that can be emotionally disturbing and sometimes scary, especially when there may be no words to describe what you are experiencing in the moment.

As in psychodynamic psychotherapy, your EMDR therapist considers childhood history and how it has contributed to your health or dysfunction. Also, during the EMDR process of desensitization you are encouraged to free associate images, thoughts, emotions, and sensations, and to accept whatever arises from the unconscious as a manifestation of the body as well as the mind. All such communication is considered potentially valuable. Some clients even use symbolism to represent their trauma. As in CBT, EMDR takes into account your conditioned responses, especially where this concerns the experience of trauma. The process of EMDR allows your negative beliefs to naturally process until a present-day positive perspective replaces them. You are then freed from beliefs that limit your life and relationships. When integrated in body-centered therapy, all this results in changes in the body (physical symptoms of trauma disappear or are greatly alleviated) and in the mind (uncontrollable emotions diminish and negative self-beliefs associated with the trauma are transformed). By acknowledging all aspects of a person's being, and by trusting in a client's process as expressed in and through the body-mind, EMDR offers healing for trauma that is more holistic and complete than other therapies.

EMDR therapy begins when your therapist guides you to find a strong picture of what the trauma represents. It is the worst part of the experience, memory, issue, or symptom. The detail of the picture is highlighted to help activate the memory network. You are then guided to scan inside to feel the negative beliefs, emotions, and related body sensations associated with the picture. Always your therapist will guide you to keep in close touch with whatever arises, whether it be new images, thoughts, emotions, or physical sensations. Each person has his or her own unique way of processing. Some people may see or hear things; some may find the mind fills with many thoughts; some may feel the mind and body full of emotions; or some may sense physical sensations in the body. It's your therapist's responsibility to observe your body's most minute shifts and changes, monitor your progress, and guide you whenever necessary to facilitate the process. EMDR as an integrative therapy allows you to experience healing and know that real change can occur.

Research is showing that people who suffer from PTSD experience more activation in the limbic region of the brain and that traditional talk therapies do not appear to help a person keep from exhibiting a conditioned body response. You can try to talk yourself out of a reaction, but that is almost impossible. The nonverbal response happens so quickly that understanding of what is happening in the present moment doesn't change the reaction (van der Kolk, 1994). You may have insight, but changing the reaction has to come from a different kind of therapy.

Research is also showing that EMDR is more effective than many other types of trauma therapies. This has been demonstrated through at least 20 controlled (16 published) studies testing the efficacy of EMDR as a treatment for PTSD. (More may be completed after this writing that could be found at www.emdria.org.) The studies have consistently shown the superiority of EMDR over other types of trauma therapies. A study financed by Kaiser Permanente revealed that EMDR was twice as effective in half the amount of time as the standard traditional care. Comparative studies included biofeedback relaxation (Carlson et al., 1998), active listening (Scheck et al., 1998), standard care (group therapy) in a Veterans Administration hospital (Boudewyns & Hyer, 1996), and standard care (various forms of individual therapy) in a Kaiser HMO facility (Marcus, Marquis, & Sakai, 1997).

There have also been clinical trials comparing CBT to EMDR. These results have been mixed and show that EMDR and CBT both have good results with their respective treatments of PTSD. Some found CBT superior to EMDR (Devilly & Spence, 1999) while others found EMDR superior (Ironson et al., 2002; Power et al., 2002). The last reported study showed that even when the therapeutic results were comparable, treatment with EMDR required fewer sessions than CBT, a potential savings to the client of both time and money.

CHAPTER SIX

EMDR for Children

The best and most beautiful things in the world cannot be seen or even touched. They must be felt within the heart.

Helen Keller

I get asked all the time if EMDR works for children, and the answer is yes. EMDR is great for helping children reprocess trauma. Often children's behaviors and emotional issues are rooted in some kind of trauma that parents may not know about. It may be big-T traumas, or many times it's little-t traumas. School, peers, and fitting in can be overwhelming for children. When they start struggling emotionally and behaviorally, if disturbing events were involved it's good to clear those memories with EMDR so that the child can be more present, feel more confident, and cope better in all areas of life.

If you're looking for an EMDR therapist for your child, be sure to ask if the therapist specializes in working with children and is qualified in EMDR. Usually, the therapist will begin by working with you, the parents. The therapist will rely on you to describe your child's problem, either over the phone or in person, so that the therapist can give an expert opinion about whether EMDR might be helpful. If the therapist does think it might help, you will be given an explanation of EMDR, much as I have provided in this book. The therapist will take a history from you in order to get some idea about what is going on in your child's life. Unless your child is old enough to participate and wants to be involved, this first history-taking session will be with you alone. You will be asked all those nosy questions I talked about earlier in the book, along with some additional personal information about both parents if your therapist thinks it is relevant to treatment. If there are any medical or psychiatric issues involving the child (illnesses, medications, and such), your therapist may ask your permission to speak to the medical providers, both to inform them that your child will be doing therapy and to get their opinion about what's going on. If there are any legal issues involving the child or child custody, your therapist may ask to consult with the lawyer involved before proceeding with EMDR treatment. (More details about this issue can be found in Chapter 6 under Legal Issues.)

The process of EMDR is similar yet different when working with children. The principles are the same, but the execution changes because children's brains are still developing and they process trauma differently than adults. What can take an adult an hour to process can take a child 5 minutes. EMDR is usually simple with children. The child doesn't have to do anything and changes happen quickly, naturally, and smoothly. EMDR is integrated easily into other forms of therapy used with children such as talk therapy, play therapy, sand tray therapy, and art therapy. Many therapists who work with children will use an integrative approach to EMDR therapy.

Your child's therapist probably will not describe EMDR in detail to your child because it is too complicated and sophisticated for most children to comprehend. They will instead find a simple way, using the child's level of vocabulary, to explain the process of EMDR. There are, however, some teenagers and precocious kids who really want to know what you intend to do, and why, and in that case it's always a good idea to treat them as you would an adult, even if they may not fully understand what you're talking about. Depending on the age of your child, the language your therapist uses during sessions will be appropriate for your child's development. Just as with adults, the treatment will begin with resourcing. The therapist will help your child find a safe place, usually an easy process for children because their imaginations are not yet restricted. If necessary (and it usually is) your child will be taught self-soothing techniques.

Your child will be introduced to BLS. BLS with children can be done with eye movements, pulsers, hand taps, playing patty cake with the therapist, drumming, or even stomping feet. Again, the right way to do it is simply what works best for your child.

The therapist will also help your child learn to put the disturbing issues or feelings away in a container. Again, this often proves easier with imaginative children than self-conscious adults (although, of course, hyper-self-conscious teenagers will often feel that this kind of exercise is silly). Many children will be instructed to write or draw the bad stuff on pieces of paper. Then the paper containing all the distress is put in an envelope that they can open it up later to be worked on another day. This teaches them the skill of containment. In a kind of feedback loop, therapists who work with children tend to get more creative when exposed to children's imaginative flexibility and creativity through the therapeutic process.

When building targets, the age of the child will be taken into consideration and the protocol, as needed, will be modified during the setup. While research about child development has taught us a great deal about what is age appropriate for children, each child is unique in his or her development and so how the therapist sets up the session will depend on the assessment of your child. Children above the age of 12 will probably be able to find a strong image, a negative belief, a positive belief, and be able to rate the positive belief as well as identify emotions and rate the level of disturbance and track this in their bodies. When children are younger than age 12, the therapist will have to take into account the child's capabilities in creating the target. Some children can identify a strong image and beliefs while others can't. Whatever the situation, the therapist will adapt EMDR to the needs of your child so that he or she feels comfortable and the process has the best possibility of success. Sometimes therapists use pictures to help children express emotions and the degree of upset they feel. Or the therapist might ask your child to show with his hands how big his upset is. While such adaptations may seem simplistic and awkward on this page, in sessions they are usually smooth, easy, and effective.

When your child begins the desensitization phase, the therapist will use a method of BLS. Children under age 6 will more likely use hand taps. Eye movement might be too difficult because their eye coordination hasn't fully developed yet. When working with very young children, a therapist may use words that are believed to reflect emotional upset for the child such as *hurt*, *bad*, or *big*. These words are intended to activate the child's memory network. Sometimes the therapist will tell the whole traumatic story of what happened to the child while the child is processing with BLS. Sometimes, if appropriate, a parent may be asked to hold the child and tell the traumatic story while BLS is applied. As you can see, what's important is that EMDR occur in a setting where the child feels comfortable and safe.

Once the desensitization is complete, the natural process will be to move into the installation phase, where the child will establish and reinforce positive beliefs and emotions. With children this may look a little different than with adults. The therapist may have to prompt a child—"So, what do you think now?"—and accept a "happy statement" rather than a specific positive belief. Such happy statements tend to spontaneously arise from children during the process.

As with adults, a session will always end in a way that makes your child feel safe and protected. This will happen whether the processing has been completed or not. Your child's therapist may use a safe place or other modalities to help soothe your child. The therapist will probably suggest that the parents monitor their child's progress between sessions at home. Any changes in behaviors or symptoms should be reported to the therapist in the following session. The therapist will always recheck the work in the next session to see if processing was truly completed. If not, then the processing of the previous issue will continue. If it was processed fully, then the child will move on to the next issue. When working with children it's important to emphasize that the memory is not going to go away, only the disturbing feelings and sensations they experience when they remember the traumatic event.

Here are some symptoms that may suggest that EMDR could be helpful to your child. Initially, your therapist may work with the child's responses or traumas, trying to help alleviate some of the symptoms by building skills and resources. As these are generalities and there are many possible causes, always be sure to consult with your physician as well as with a qualified EMDR therapist before involving your child in EMDR therapy.

- Anxiety and fear such as school phobia.
- Nightmares and night terrors.
- Persistent bed wetting.
- Unreasonable or excessive guilt.
- Anger and tantrums.
- Depression.
- Some medical issues (depending on cause and symptoms).
- Epilepsy—your therapist may want to talk to your child's

physician before starting EMDR. EMDR has been used with children who experience epilepsy with success. EMDR will not cure epilepsy but may possibly help with the traumatic feelings of being different.

- Hallucinations (depending on cause and symptoms).
- Oppositional behavior.
- Dissociation.
- Hyperactivity.
- Academic difficulties.
- Developmental delay.
- Learning disorders—it can be traumatic for an individual to feel different when they have a learning disorder. Again, EMDR will not heal the learning disorder, but may help with the traumatic feelings.

Even if your child is struggling in a current traumatic situation (the slow death of a grandparent, for example), studies are now finding that EMDR can help build resiliency and give the child the ability to cope more effectively and with less upset in future difficult situations.

There are times, of course, when EMDR may not be helpful for your child. As a parent, you should discuss this with your child's physician and prospective EMDR therapist for their expert advice about the best treatment plan.

Children 12 and Older

With a child over the age of 12, it is especially important for the therapist to validate the child's experience and assess if he or she is comfortable with the therapist. If not, then regardless of the therapist's professional qualifications, it's advisable to interview a couple of therapists to find the right one for your child. Remember, the most important indicator of successful therapy is the relationship between the client and the therapist.

At this age, the parents usually come to the first visit so that everyone can hear what EMDR is about and get a clear idea about what to expect. The parents then leave the room so that work can begin with the child. EMDR can be especially effective for teenagers who find it difficult to reveal too much of their story. It's easier for teens to come to therapy if they don't have to share too much information about their trauma. The first session will probably be spent on resourcing, finding a safe place and a container. Some therapists might also teach some of the other preparation skills like relaxation and breathing. The therapist may also find what experiences make the client feel good about himself or herself and build on those resources. If the child is ready, processing may begin in the next session.

The following is a case example of how EMDR helped a 15-year-old girl get her life back on track.

Sandy

Sandy was a high school student who came for EMDR therapy because she was skipping classes at school. Her parents were starting to worry about her. Sandy's parents had divorced when she was young and her mother later married a man with whom Sandy didn't get along. Academically, Sandy was a bright student, but recently her grades had begun to drop. Her parents discovered that she'd started smoking pot with her friends and they were concerned about how this was affecting her grades. They also noticed that she seemed more depressed, wasn't sleeping well, and was losing her appetite. Her mother called and shared this over the phone along with more of Sandy's history.

After the therapist talked to Sandy's parents and explained the EMDR process, the parents agreed to go ahead with treatment. When meeting with Sandy, it was important for her to feel that her story was important and that she could get help. When asked, "What's the most upsetting thing that's ever happened to you?" Sandy opened up a little about how badly her peers had treated her. It was incredibly humiliating when they teased her. This suggested a first target for EMDR.

Sandy's first session began with finding her safe place. She imagined waking in a country field that felt open and free. She then worked on her container and imagined a beautifully painted box that she could close and lock. It was also noted that Sandy liked basketball and when playing felt good, strong, and competent. This resource was important because Sandy was able to feel something positive. Sandy successfully used BLS to strengthen these positive states, indicating that she was ready to begin her EMDR desensitization.

Sandy decided that she liked the pulsers for the BLS and for her stop sign she would raise her hand. The first target needed to be assessed. She wanted to work on not feeling like she fit in with the other kids. She felt the kids were mean to her and that they judged everything she did. Here was the assessment for the target:

- Image: "Those girls making fun of my clothes and calling me names. They are standing there with these awful looking faces and I feel like an outcast."
- Negative belief: "I'm stupid."
- Positive belief: "I can be a good student and have friends."
- VoC scale: "2."
- Emotions: "Sad, angry."
- SUDS scale: "7."
- Location of body sensation: "All over my body."

Sandy's sessions were 60 minutes long, half talk and half processing with EMDR. The first session went quickly. She was able to bring up the image, feel "stupid," feel sad and angry, and experience this throughout her body. She easily signaled that she was ready for BLS to begin. The first set went quickly. She was quiet during the processing until she yawned, which was an indication to stop the BLS and check in. During the set, she remembered feeling embarrassed and then realized that she was angry at her friends. The anger went away quickly and then her mind wandered off to thinking about shopping at the mall after the session. Another set of BLS began and then stopped after a short period of time. She said that she had felt really angry at her friends and then right after that the anger dissipated. Her mind wandered again to going shopping at the mall. She was processing rapidly. With another set she said that she wasn't angry anymore. She just wished people would be nicer to her. During that set she moved more in the chair as if she was anxious. That experience seemed to move through very fast also. Her mind drifted off to the mall again. Another set of BLS was completed. She wished that she had more friends. Through the desensitization phase she processed more until she spontaneously started remembering the good times she had at camp over the summer and how wonderful the people were to her. This was the resource within her naturally coming forward, helping her remember more positive times in her life. The desensitization was checked for completion and nothing else was connected to this event that could be disturbing. Her positive cognition changed to "I'm okay and I do have some friends." Sandy worked with that until she completely believed it and felt strong and more confident.

Then her present triggers were assessed and processed. Her biggest fear was going to school the next day. This scenario was processed thoroughly until Sandy could feel good about going to school without feeling upset or any disturbance. More resources came up as she processed. She spontaneously concluded with the statement, "I can handle whatever comes up. I'm a good student. I have friends."

Sandy's body relaxed and she felt like she had more energy. Her work was complete for this session. The session ended with a body scan and closure just as they do for adults. You can see in this session how quickly the processing occurred. Children can move through these kinds of issues much faster than adults. Sandy resolved this incident rapidly and found new strengths from within. She went to school the next day with a new sense of confidence and ease.

When working with teenagers, it's important to help them find their strengths and do resource development to support and enhance those strengths. This helps teens realize that they are more than their troubles. Because Sandy had success with her first target, she was able to proceed to the next target in the following session: processing her parents' divorce. Divorce is always difficult for kids and many times they have no one with whom they can share their feelings. Often they end up repressing their feelings and then act out later in their lives. Although she sensed that this would be difficult, Sandy felt that she was ready and trusted EMDR and her therapist enough to go forward.

During the divorce Sandy was unable to turn to her mother because her mother had been so emotionally upset and un-available. She successfully processed her feelings about this and came to her third session ready to deal with the anger she felt toward her stepfather. This, too, processed easily.

During these three weeks of sessions, Sandy's mood greatly improved. During the next two she decided she needed to change high schools because it was too difficult to return to the school with all the bad memories. She decided this on her own and her parents honored that decision because they wanted to support the change in their daughter. Once in her new school, she started making new friends, eating better, and sleeping better. She said that she felt more comfortable in her own skin. Seven months later she checked in. She was doing well, wasn't smoking pot, had great friends, and was participating in sports.

In five sessions, Sandy was able to process her anxiety and depression, and find more inner confidence and strength knowing that she could change her life. With the support of her parents, she was able to move through some little-t traumas that were affecting her emotionally and behaviorally with the help of EMDR.

Children Ages 7–11

When children are between the ages of 7 and 11, the parents are sometimes invited into the room during processing to help the child feel safer, if appropriate and if the parents have the skills to do this. The parents are frequently traumatized vicariously by their child's trauma. As the parents visually watch their child progress and get better and better, the parents begin to relax, which in turn helps the child heal. This can benefit everyone. Sometimes, though, the parents may need to do their own EMDR in order to help support the family system.

The therapy begins, as usual, with finding a safe place. It might be necessary to develop containment, too, but for many children it's not necessary because they process the trauma so quickly that there's nothing left to be contained. This work can often take less than three sessions to complete. Of course, if there are more complicated family issues involving more traumas, the therapy can take longer.

Next is a case example of a 9-year-old boy who suffered immensely until he processed his trauma with EMDR.

Chris

Chris came into therapy for EMDR because of a horrible bike accident. While he was biking one day with friends, they got separated. Going downhill, he lost control of his bike. He fell hard and rolled several times, breaking his right leg. He didn't remember much other than that someone must have called the police. He remembered that he was hurt badly, felt all alone, and was frightened by the strange people surrounding him. The ambulance was scary and his body felt frozen. When his parents met him at the hospital it was a huge relief. The doctors put a cast on his leg but later discovered that it wasn't healing properly. They were going to have to break his leg again and reset it. This operation added to the original trauma of the accident because he wasn't given enough anesthesia during the operation. He woke up during the surgery and, completely aware but unable to move or speak, "freaked out."

About a year after the accident, his leg was healing but he was suffering from headaches and stomachaches, didn't want to go to school anymore, felt anxious when left alone, and wasn't sleeping well. He was also dreading yet another surgery in a couple of months to remove some screws in his leg.

This trauma began with a single incident, but later events were just as painful for Chris. All the pieces of the traumatic experience needed to be processed with EMDR. Chris's life was being affected to the extent that he was barely functioning. His mother brought him in for therapy wondering if EMDR could help. His fear level was high and so his mother stayed in the room during the sessions.

Therapy began with Chris finding a safe place. Chris loved to draw and for his safe place drew his favorite room of the house, the family room, watching TV with his parents by his side. For his BLS he liked the Tac/Audio Scan, using the earphones.

The first target was the accident. Each piece of the trauma after the accident would also be worked on so that Chris could integrate and transform this horrible event. Here is the assessment of the target:

- Image: "Looking down and seeing my leg doesn't look right."
- Negative belief: "I'm bad."
- Positive belief: "I am good."
- VoC scale: "2."
- Emotions: "Scared, My leg looks creepy."
- SUDS scale: "10."
- Location of body sensation: "Chest and leg."

When Chris was fully connected to this memory, the BLS started. Chris immediately began to process the difficult feelings and within a few minutes began talking about what he was having for dinner. Directed back to the image, he said that part seemed to be fine. He then identified the next disturbing image of waking up during the surgery. He got in touch with the associated emotions, the BLS started, and he began to process. Within minutes he started talking about the book he was currently reading. Brought back to the surgery image, he said it didn't bother him. This process continued, going step by step through the entire sequence of events up until the current day. He processed and cleared nine different images during the session. At the end of the session, his SUDS level was checked on the original target and it had decreased to a level of 3. He was then instructed to go to his safe place to end the session.

In his second session Chris reported that his SUDS had gone back up to a 5. This can happen in EMDR because the work has not been completed. The image of his weird-looking leg still bothered him. He processed that image again with BLS. He was instructed to tell the whole story from beginning to end. Everything felt clear except, again, the image of his crooked, busted leg, which remained at a SUDS 5. This time while processing his therapists asked him to look at his leg while he was seeing the disturbing image in his mind's eye. He could see that his leg was fine, and this physical truth set him free. The SUDS dropped immediately to a 0. His positive belief changed to "I'm fine and my leg is fine." This positive self-belief was paired with the memory of the traumatic event and installed using BLS until it was a VoC of 7.

In his third session, Chris's mother reported that he was sleeping well, participating in sports, and for the first time since the accident he got back on his bike and rode for hours with no anxiety.

Finally, Chris worked on his anxiety about the forthcoming

surgery. His mother researched information about what they could expect, talked to his doctor, and even took Chris to the hospital. Still, he felt anxious. This time he told the story of what had happened out loud while processing with the BLS. He talked about and processed each step of the past surgery, which would also be each step of the upcoming surgery: preparing for the surgery at home, going to the hospital, being prepped in the hospital, anesthesia. When this was complete, Chris was instructed to visualize the upcoming event from beginning to end while using the BLS to help process the future fear and anxiety. The disturbing feelings cleared completely.

His mother took him again for a visit to the hospital and reported that Chris felt no anxiety about the upcoming surgery. He felt confident he could handle it and he would be okay. Chris did his self-care routine everyday, listening to his favorite music, which he said soothed him. He often used his safe place to calm himself on a regular basis from the stresses of school. As a side benefit, as Chris worked through this trauma his mom felt her own anxiety lessen because she no longer had to worry so much about her child. Chris was able to go through the surgery with less fear, more confidence, and believing that no matter what he would be okay.

Children Ages 0–5

EMDR can even help young children of the 0–5 age range process traumatic events that they are struggling to assimilate. Often therapists will use other modalities of therapy to facilitate EMDR processing, since the children may not be able to voice all that they are feeling. This can involve a variety of forms. To access a target for a child of this age, the therapist may talk about the traumatic event to stimulate the child's memory network. Some therapists have the child draw the traumatic event as well as his feelings about it. If the therapist uses sand tray therapy, the child can create a story with characters that represent the traumatic event. Or, if the child can't describe the trauma, the therapist may invite the parents to tell the story, making sure the story ends with everything being okay, including the child, and Mommy and Daddy. Once the target is assessed through whatever method the therapist is trained in, BLS is added to facilitate the processing.

The entire process is about establishing safety for the child, activating the traumatic memory however possible, processing in the most feasible way, and then always ending with a reaffirmation of safety. Because children's brains do not associate memories the way mature brains do, the process can prove much easier and faster for them than for adults. EMDR processing is adapted to the ability of the child so that healing can occur naturally.

CHAPTER SEVEN

Safety Measures for EMDR

Life was meant to be lived, and curiosity must be kept alive.
One must never, for whatever reason, turn his back on life.

Eleanor Roosevelt

People often ask me if EMDR will help them. In many cases the answer is yes. If you have experienced a big-T trauma, EMDR is great for moving through the pain of that event. If you have experienced little-t trauma, EMDR can often be helpful, although the treatment may take longer. Some clients need to slow down and spend more time in the preparation phase to make it feel safer to eventually move into the reprocessing phase. If someone has spent years not feeling their feelings and is defended in such a way that the feelings aren't accessible, then EMDR isn't the right therapy until they can learn to access their feelings. Talk therapy as well as body-centered therapies are appropriate to learn these skills.

Also, therapy takes commitment and work. I assign most of my clients homework, consisting of practicing safe place and containment, deep breathing, and relaxation. The clients who benefit most from therapy are those willing to do the work and commit to the process. Some clients will need to practice what they have learned until it becomes second nature and then integrate their new way of being into the world, while others will just resolve their traumas and move on quickly.

Occasionally, your therapist may recommend that you not do EMDR desensitization. Reasons vary but here are a few.

Legal Issues

If you are a victim of a crime and will be involved in a court case, it is important for your therapist to know this information. This could include sexual abuse, rape, assault, auto accidents, work-related issues, and anything related to contested custody of children. Your therapist will need to talk to your lawyer to see what is involved in your case, if you will need to testify, and when that may occur. Your therapist will need to inform your lawyer about what EMDR is and the effects of the treatment. Remember, EMDR affects how vivid a memory can feel to you, so that when you think of the traumatic event the emotional charge has lessened and the memory may change. You, your lawyer, and your therapist might need to decide the best course of action for your case and treatment. If EMDR will be used, your therapist will give you a form to sign titled "Informed Consent for Eye Movement Desensitization and Reprocessing." This form will state the nature of EMDR, how memories can change from the process, and that you are consenting to this form of treatment. If it is not appropriate to do EMDR right in the beginning, resource development skills can help you in dealing with the effects of the trauma and preparing for your court proceedings.

It is important to note that in the state of Washington a legal precedent has been set that a witness who has been hypnotized will be disqualified from testifying. When memories are retrieved through hypnosis, the law does not hold these memories valid and admissible. EMDR may be viewed the same way even though it is not hypnosis. Sometimes memories will arise during an EMDR session and these memories, also, might not be admissible in court. Memories are not like video recorders. You don't hit the rewind button and watch an exact version of the event appear. Over time memories can become distorted through the association process.

Research psychologist Dr. Elizabeth Loftus has devoted her life to the study of memory. She has spent years conducting laboratory studies on the malleability of memory. She believes that "our memories are flexible and superimposable, a panoramic blackboard with an endless supply of chalk and erasers" (Loftus & Ketcham, 1994, p. 3). She has concluded from her studies that memory is not accurate. She began her research because of an experience she had when she was a child. When she was 14, she experienced a false memory. She could remember many details surrounding the death of her mother, who drowned in a swimming pool, but not the actual death. A relative told her years later that she was the one who had found her mother's body in the pool. Loftus could not remember any of this at first, and then she started remembering details of seeing her mother dead in the pool. Knowing this information, she felt at peace with all of her feelings surrounding the death. Then three days later, her uncle told her that she remembered this story wrong and it was actually her aunt who had discovered the body. The power of the suggestion overwhelmed her and has propelled her to question the accuracy of memory ever since.

Through her studies she has found that people do remember more details of traumatic events when the shock value is higher. As stated in an earlier chapter, the stronger the imprint, the stronger the memory. She also found that when people are told stories over and over, the details they remember can easily change. They will incorporate those details as the truth, suggesting that memory is not reliable and that through the power of suggestion information can easily be included in memory.

People have called me asking to use EMDR for memory retrieval. I do not use EMDR in this way. Memories arising during a session may or may not be the complete truth. Your therapist does not have the power to know whether or not your traumatic experiences happened the way you remember them. The best way to know the truth about what happened is if you have corroboration from other sources. You may uncover parts of a trauma through EMDR, but some aspects can be lost or remembered inaccurately. Your memories can be distorted over time and details can be lost. It is not necessary to remember all aspects of a trauma for you to heal from the afteraffects. What we know for sure is that your body-mind is holding some kind of trauma and this is what is being healed with EMDR. Then you will notice the change in your whole way of looking at yourself and at what has happened, and find relief for your symptoms.

Medical Issues

If you have any kind of eye condition, are on medication, or have a head injury or a heart condition, you will want to report that to your therapist during the history-taking phase. Your therapist may want to contact your physician to make sure it will be safe for you to experience EMDR therapy. Once your physician has given the go ahead, you and your therapist will determine the type of BLS that will work best for you.

Migraines

If you are a migraine sufferer, you need to let your therapist know. EMDR is not a problem if you are not currently experiencing a migraine. If you begin to experience a migraine during your session, your therapist will not do EMDR desensitization because the process could increase your pain.

Pregnancy

There is no current research on the impact of EMDR on the fetus and the issue is currently being debated among EMDR therapists. So it is up to you and your therapist to determine what is right for you until research can prove what the actual impact is on the fetus. I think it is better to be cautious and use EMDR only in relationship to issues impacting your current pregnancy that could support better bonding or a better birth process. I don't recommend processing old childhood trauma until after the baby is born.

Psychotropic Medications

If you are experiencing a major psychosis or a major depression, your therapist will not use EMDR lest the process exacerbate the problem. Once you are stable, after your therapist consults with your psychiatrist, EMDR may be possible. You can do EMDR while on psychotropic medication as long as you are stable enough to do the work and have a support system that can keep you on track with your therapy and your meds. Some medications will allow you to do the work needed for EMDR, while others may make it more difficult for you to connect to your emotions. If you process trauma while on medication, should you recover sufficiently that you no longer need medication, your therapist will probably want to go back and recheck all the targets you cleared to see if any more material arises once you're off the medication.

Alcohol and Street Drugs

Generally, it is not a good idea to do EMDR while using alcohol or street drugs. Some therapists will work with you during addiction, but they must be qualified and know what they are doing. You should never come to treatment under the influence of any substance, because it will hinder your work. Your therapist will help you build strength through good resourcing and finding new coping mechanisms for your own safety. A good support system is important, including getting involved in a 12-step group like Alcoholics Anonymous, Rational Recovery, religious organizations, or women's or men's groups, and turning to family and friends for help. If you're struggling with an addiction, I highly recommend that you deal with the addiction before EMDR or work with a therapist who specializes in addiction recovery and EMDR.

Suicidal or Homicidal

Your therapist will need to know if you are suicidal or homicidal at any point in the work you are doing. If that's how you're feeling, it's not a time to be doing deep trauma work. Trauma work might make you feel more vulnerable and out of control. The first goal in therapy is to keep you safe, and if you are suicidal or homicidal then you are not safe. This is, instead, a time to regroup, get the treatment you need, and find your strengths. Tell your therapist if you have suicidal or homicidal thoughts or plans so that she can help you find the help that you need.

Too Much Going on in Your Life

As your therapist is getting to know you, he will be looking for what is happening in your life week to week. Is your life stable enough to do this kind of work? Sometimes after sessions clients can feel drained and exhausted and might need to have some down time. If you have a test the next day or are in the process of moving, tell your therapist so that he can assess whether EMDR is a good idea for that day. Even if EMDR may not be right for you now, it might be down the road when your life calms down and you feel more settled.

PART II
Transformational Stories

Enjoy your own life without comparing it with that of another.

Marquis de Condorcet

CHAPTER EIGHT

Regaining Control After a Childhood Traumatic Event: Mary

Every wall is a door.

Ralph Waldo Emerson

When children experience a big-T trauma, it can severely hinder their development. As they grow into adulthood, they can remain stuck at the emotional age when the trauma occurred. Irrational beliefs can develop along with PTSD symptoms such as hypervigilance, feeling unsafe in the world, an inability to relax, an exaggerated startle response, nightmares, insomnia, irritation, anger, or a constant sense of stress—the list can go on and on. If the trauma is not processed at the time it occurred in childhood, then it can haunt the adult the child becomes. If the adult can't remember the trauma, she may conclude that because she's felt this way for so many years, it must be normal. It's not. Such an adult perceives the world through the filter of the trauma she experienced as a child and often reacts to her world as if the trauma is happening over and over again. Her body-mind imbalance may lead to forms of depression, anxiety, or hopelessness. It may also show up in difficulties in relationships, and often she may attempt to self-medicate with legal or illegal drugs.

You'll remember that a big-T trauma is defined as an event

that is perceived as horrific and life threatening, with a sense of helplessness prevailing. EMDR can be helpful to someone who experienced this kind of traumatic event as a child. EMDR processes the past childhood trauma into new and healthier, more adaptive thoughts and behaviors as an adult.

Mary was 36 and had been married for 8 years when she came to see me for treatment of extreme anxiety. Not only was she anxious, she felt on the verge of losing control most of the time and was also uncomfortable with people and easily startled by stimuli in her environment. She felt constantly tense and had become increasingly fearful—of what, she couldn't say exactly; she just didn't feel safe. A therapist friend had suggested she give EMDR a try and she had come despite some reservations.

Mary was an attractive woman but looked uncomfortable in her own skin. When she first appeared in therapy, I worried that she was so disconnected from her body that she wasn't even aware that she had one. As she told me about her situation, she raced through her stories, jumping from point to point very quickly. She had so much to share that it felt as if she was about ready to burst if she didn't get everything out all at once. Her anxiety was so intense that it was hard for her to sit still on the couch. She looked as if she was ready to launch into the rest of her day and that sitting with me was torture. As she was racing verbally, she told me that her husband wanted to have children but she didn't; she felt she didn't deserve to be a mother. Mary had developed a fear of being a parent.

Mary also revealed that she felt a deep need to help animals, although she didn't know why; she thought that her grandmother's love of animals must have influenced her. She kept picking up stray animals, many with disabilities. At one point she'd adopted six cats. It upset her to the point of "torture" if she saw any animal suffering and she felt it her duty to rescue those in need of help. She suffered from insomnia, and when she did sleep she often had nightmares that woke her. By the time I saw her, these symptoms had gone on for years. She was tired and knew something was wrong but had no idea why she felt so horrible. Even though she recognized that there were some good things in her current life, she had trouble feeling positive. She was desperate and didn't know if getting to the bottom of what was causing her such distress could really help relieve her PTSD symptoms.

As we explored her history, Mary revealed that her parents had divorced when she was young, that after the divorce her father left and she'd felt abandoned, that her brother had had cancer but survived, and that her grandfather had also died when she was young (she still vividly remembered seeing him ill). Her mother then married a man with whom Mary didn't connect. She felt unseen in her family and restricted from being the person she wanted to be. She held herself in check all the time and often heard a highly critical voice inside her own mind telling her that she was bad and a horrible person. The voice seemed to have a distinct power over her. She could not control it and it disturbed her to the point that she often felt crazy.

Over a couple of weeks, as Mary shared more of her family history, she eventually remembered an event at age 9 that clearly had much to do with her fear and her sense that she didn't deserve to be a mother. She had forgotten this memory but during the process of getting to know her the memory came flooding back and she shared it with me. When she was a child she lived on an island where animals were starving, including cats and dogs. An 18-year-old friend had a cat that was pregnant, and she told Mary that the kittens wouldn't be able to live. One night after the kittens were born, her friend asked Mary to help euthanize them. Why her friend asked for help from a 9-year-old, Mary didn't know. Mary was reluctant, but when she arrived and found her friend sobbing, she decided to help. She sensed that this wasn't right but also didn't want the kittens to suffer. Mary remembered feeling calm but now realized that in fact she'd moved out of her body and was numb. Her friend planned to use ether, and Mary thought it would be like in the movies; put a piece of cloth over the kittens' mouths and they would gently go to sleep. Instead, the kittens struggled, shrieked, and bled from their noses. Mary was shocked, and then appalled when she realized that her desperate friend planned to bury the kittens, dead or alive. She fled and suppressed this memory. Remembering this experience, she heard an inner voice tell her, "If you are capable of murdering infant animals then you're evil and don't deserve to be a parent; you can't be trusted." Mary's fears had become her penance. She believed that there was no atoning for killing the kittens and she must suffer for the rest of her life. Now it was clear why she was constantly rescuing animals and being so reactive.

I knew that we would have to do EMDR to help Mary resolve the horror of this past event and set her free of the guilt and pain she'd held inside for so long. But first we had to develop her resources so that she could deal with the emotions that were bound to arise. As she kept sharing her history, we developed some resources to help her feel better in her present life and to give her better coping skills to deal with her extreme symptoms of PTSD.

Mary struggled to find a safe place. Because she couldn't ever remember feeling a sense of safety, we changed the language and called it a relaxed place. Helping her experience and recognize a relaxed feeling in her body-mind was challenging. Her mind raced with many negative thoughts and her body was used to bracing against danger and threat. I guided her gently to sit and become mindful of the sensations she felt in her body. I asked her to track only one sensation at a time, just to notice without having to change or fix anything. Slowly, she began to develop the ability to sit and be with her physical sensations while watching as her mind tried to judge the sensations as wrong, bad, or scary. Doing this practice, she found a way to observe the critical voice from a distance so that she could sit with her physical experience and notice that in the present moment she was okay and safe.

One day Mary arrived for her session and told me that she experienced a pleasant feeling at her office one day. The sun was shining through the window and she could feel the warmth on her skin. Her resources were beginning to build; she'd found some relaxation along with a positive feeling. We brought up her relaxed place and added eye movement as her BLS to support the image and feelings of this experience. Although at first Mary could tolerate only very short sets of BLS before her mind raced to negative judgments, this quickly changed and she was able to sustain more BLS with her relaxed place.

We also worked on developing a container for her disturbing thoughts and feelings. Over and over she tried to come up with an image, until finally she could imagine a wall that was strong enough to hold the bad thoughts far enough away from her that she could feel some separation from them.

Mary also needed to get reacquainted with her body. She was disconnected most of the time and felt only the hypervigilance of anxiety that had become such a familiar burden that it felt normal to her. I taught her deep belly breathing and progressive relaxation; tensing her muscles on each inhale, then relaxing her muscles on each exhale. She decided to take dance classes and get regular massages so that she could become more aware of her body and its holding patterns. As she continued to see me, we strengthened her relaxed place and her container while I also educated her about what was, from a healthy adult perspective, appropriate and inappropriate for a child's development. A couple of sessions later, Mary was ready to do EMDR. With Mary's determination and commitment to her process, we both felt she was ready to begin clearing some trauma.

We decided that the euthanasia of the kittens was the first target to work on in order to help her find some resolution to this old horror. She chose eye movement for her BLS. Her stop signal was closing her eyes to cue me if she needed to stop processing. We assessed her first target.

- Worst image: "I'm in the room with the shrieking kittens."
- Negative belief: "I'm evil."
- Positive belief: "I was just a kid and I forgive myself."
- VoC scale: "1."
- Emotions: "Agony, suffering, anxiety, fear, confusion, shock, numbness, and horror."
- SUDS scale: "10."
- Location of body sensation: "Constriction in my throat, pain in my heart, pressure in my upper chest, tension in my esophagus, and difficulty breathing."

We worked together on her target memory through four sessions. These were difficult and painful for her. Many times she felt overwhelmed by the pain, but she was able to stay with the process. At times other memories would surface while she worked on her target, memories that were linked by association to the traumatic event with the kittens, such as the illness of her brother, the death of her grandfather, and almost drowning in a scuba diving accident. All of these traumas were linked to the issue of death and dying. When this happened I'd guide her to allow these associative memories to rise into consciousness and unwind, like watching a movie, as BLS helped her brain recall, reprocess, and release events that had haunted her for so long. Working with these memories, she came to realize that she was afraid to go to sleep at night out of fear that she might die and never wake up again. She also realized that because she believed she was such a horrible person and was unable to forgive herself, her self-tortures in the form of her symptoms were far worse than anything anyone else would subject her to.

Like many clients, as she focused intently on the target memory, Mary was surprised to discover how this event and her traumatic reaction to it had become a template for her life as it unfolded through other traumatic events, all of which contributed to her anxiety and the sense that her life was out of her control.

But difficult as it was, Mary persevered, and as we worked through that first horrific memory, things began to change. Gradually, as she felt more connected to her body, and able to tolerate disturbing emotions and allow them to move through her body-mind, she began to trust that she was going to be all right. Her physical tension, level of anxiety, and hypervigilance all decreased. She believed that she could handle daily events with less stress and felt more in control of her life.

By Mary's last session she reported feeling no disturbance in her body, mind, or soul. Through the work she found compassion and forgiveness for herself. She could sense her positive belief, "I was just a kid and I forgive myself." Mary continued to work on other issues in therapy, all the while living with this new belief to see how it might change her life.

Six months after Mary had completed this EMDR target, she came to my office and told me, "I get it; the EMDR is really working. The change has been happening over time; I couldn't see it so clearly in the moment. But now I can see I'm reacting differently. Even my husband can see the difference."

While Mary still feels compassion for animals, she's no longer compelled to sacrifice herself to save them; now she feels it's a choice. As her suffering has decreased, so has her anxiety. Her nightmares have stopped completely and she can sleep through the night. Her coping skills have improved and she feels more self-compassion and forgiveness. During the following 3 years of continued therapy she had two children and discovered that she's a competent mother with much to offer them. This trauma is now in the past where it belongs.

Although Mary continues to struggle with different issues

from her childhood that cause her distress as an adult, as the layers peel away she continues to trust the process and strengthen her coping skills. She realizes that the traumatic event with the kittens was just a piece of a much larger puzzle and she is committed to putting together one piece of the puzzle at a time so that she can be the best woman, wife, and mother that she can be. She now looks comfortable in her body and is committed to her EMDR journey.

CHAPTER NINE

Decreasing Anxiety by Letting Go of Control: Carolyn

We have all a better guide in ourselves, if we would attend to it, than any other person can be.

Jane Austen

Anxiety is a normal response to danger. We are programmed in our brain and nervous system to feel anxious when we sense danger coming our way. We all feel anxiety at different points of the day as the result of the pressures and stress of this fast-paced world we live in. Trying to balance home, work, and family is no easy task. While anxiety can help us avoid certain dangers—you get a gut feeling something isn't right and you act on it—feeling anxious all the time can be too much for your system and can drain you of vital energy. If you didn't feel some anxiety, there would be something wrong with you. Normal anxiety rises and falls like an emotional wave on an essentially calm sea.

When you feel anxious all the time, however, it's more like you're living through an unending series of storms and other dangers. You tend to worry all the time that something bad is going to happen, and this worry can be felt as tension throughout the body. This state becomes the norm and you don't even recognize how it's impacting your life. You end up with tight muscles, headaches, gastrointestinal problems, aches and pains, insomnia, poor concentration, irritability, and always feel tired, fatigued, and often so restless you can't sit still.

If this goes on long enough you may experience low self-esteem, depression, and obsessive thinking, and you may feel that you need to please others to make them feel okay. Sometimes you may struggle with the belief that you can't get what you want and although you always strive to be in control, you often feel that you have none. Because you look competent on the outside, the world often has no idea that you're struggling with the sense that you're falling apart on the inside. Because you spend a lot of time convincing yourself that everything's all right, it's often difficult to be specific about why you're feeling the way you feel.

Carolyn came into therapy because of her anxiety. She was a 53-year-old married mother of two children who felt anxious and hypervigilant with her 14-year-old son and wanted to feel less stressed and more "centered." Carolyn felt that she had to stay on top of everything or things would fall apart. She had difficulty letting her son lead his own life without giving unasked-for advice or trying to control his behavior. She knew this was counterproductive for him and for their relationship. She longed to trust him, to let him make his own mistakes and learn from them, but felt compelled to intervene. She could feel that her anxiety was over the top but didn't know how to effect a change.

Carolyn came into therapy looking strong and competent. She sat straight on the couch and had a sense of contained energy throughout her body. Her movements were small and tight and she clearly kept it together as she told me about her life. She kept constant eye contact and her breathing was barely visible. She had a determined look on her face as she described how she wanted things to change.

I took Carolyn's family history and learned that her father, crippled by polio, had been unable to walk. Carolyn, the middle child of three, became the self-designated responsible child who believed that without her help her family could not and would not hold together emotionally. Eventually, she got so good at being the responsible person that it seemed the normal way to be. She didn't realize that she was assuming the same role with her son that she'd assumed with her family of origin, and that this unconscious behavior was affecting her as a parent.

We began our work with calming techniques to help her cope with her anxiety. The first calming resource to put in place was her safe place. Carolyn imagined she was on the beach with the sun warming her skin and she was listening to the lapping of the ocean waves. We added BLS to enhance this calm, peaceful feeling. She was relieved that she actually could let herself have this feeling in the moment. She enjoyed her safe place so much she didn't want to come back out of it. I let her linger as long as she wanted in this space to encourage her nervous system to find some relaxation.

Next we worked on finding a container. She needed a place to put everything away that she worried about, usually a long list of tasks that hadn't been completed yet. Carolyn decided that her container was a bank vault; she would use the tumbler lock to contain her upset inside.

We then worked on deep belly breathing. I explained that this was important to help her shift from her sympathetic nervous system (fight, flee, or freeze) to her parasympathetic nervous system (rest and digest). If she could learn to slow down her breathing, her anxiety would also lessen; it might not go away entirely but would become more tolerable. She tackled this assignment like everything else in her life, but then realized that she'd have to let go some and not work so hard at it if it was really going to work.

I then asked her to pay attention to the feelings that arose when her son did something that brought on anxiety, for example, being late or not calling to check in. When she did, her pulse rose, her muscles tensed, and she said she felt out of control. I had her track the physical sensations and locate precisely where in her body she felt that feeling-sense of being out of control. When I had her stay with this feeling-sense, there arose in her mind a negative self-belief: "I'm not a good parent because he's not responsible." This caused her considerable emotional distress, so I asked her to return to her safe place. Immediately, she calmed down. We then worked on containing these upsetting emotions in her bank vault, so that she could be more present with her son and he would not feel that she was anxiously trying to control his life. I then helped her learn some simple relaxation exercises like counting to 10 and taking slow, deep breaths, the first to give her some time to focus and calm herself before responding, the second to induce calm when anxiety brought on rapid, shallow breathing. We also worked on her irrational belief that she was not a good mother. By considering her family as a whole as well as the many good and successful things her son was doing, it became clear to Carolyn that she had not failed as a mother. The truth of the matter was that she and her son had very different personalities, that how they defined responsibility was quite different, and that she would need to accept and appreciate those differences.

As Carolyn developed her skills and our trust developed, she was ready to do some EMDR. We looked at the presenting issue around her son and how anxious he made her feel. Carolyn liked the pulsers for her BLS and she would slightly raise her hand for her stop signal. We assessed the target to work on for our session. Her son had not prepared for an upcoming event, which resulted in making the whole family late. She needed him to be on time so she could feel good about him and about herself. I started with lighting up the memory network by asking a few questions.

- Image: "Being late and feeling like everyone at the event was judging me as a bad parent."
- Negative belief: "I'm a bad parent."
- Location of body sensation: "Pressure in my chest."

As she experienced the disturbance of this memory network, I asked her to just let her mind trace back to an earlier time in her life, without censoring, and tell me the first thing that came to her mind. I had a feeling this current issue was related to a past trauma from our earlier discussions and wanted to make sure we were working with the right target. This process often helps a client remember back through the memory networks to the earliest traumatic event—or what I call the root of the problem. When the root is processed, then the more current issues dissipate quickly.

This process took her to an image of her dad, unable to walk and needing her attention and assistance—attention that, as a child, she didn't always want to give, and assistance she was not always able to provide. We now had the earliest image, and together we fully assessed this target so we could process it in the desensitization phase.

- Image: "My dad unable to walk and I'm all alone."
- Negative belief: "I'm a bad person."
- Positive belief: "I'm a good person."
- VoC scale: "3."
- Emotions: "Shame, guilt, anxiety, vulnerability, and not feeling safe."
- SUDS scale: "10."
- Location of body sensation: "Increased pressure in my chest."

We began the desensitization process with the BLS. Despite the emotions and sensations she felt, Carolyn's process was internal and quiet. She showed little outward emotional response and talked very little. But there was no need for her to tell me the whole story because I could see that she was moving through it on her own. My role as a therapist was to guide her, hold a space where she would feel safe enough to have her experience, and bear witness to her healing process. After very long sets of bilateral stimulation she would check in with me, and as she did it became clear that her emotions and body sensations were becoming less disturbing, her thinking less rigidly black and white, and her self-belief more positive.

Through EMDR, Carolyn began to feel even calmer and freer, and she realized that she'd always had a deep desire for a healthy father who could have taken care of her as a child and could make her feel protected and safe in the world as she was growing up. Instead, he'd needed her to take care of him. There'd been little room for her to be a child in her family; often she felt like the parent. This realization was difficult for her to process at first and she felt tremendously guilty for even having the thought. It took her some time to realize this was the truth, her truth, and that she had to find a way to integrate this new information. We continued sets of BLS until this felt more solid and real for her.

She also realized that she felt pressure to perform and be perfect in order to keep the family stable and together. As she got older she became overly responsible, taking over the duties and responsibilities of others. She was a "wonder woman" who was stressed to the max from everything she did, and yet still felt that it was never enough, because of the underlying root belief that no matter what she did as a child, it could, in reality, never be enough for her crippled father and stressed, depressed mother. She kept trying to fix an utterly unfixable family problem. When she came to this truth, a lightbulb went off and she could finally recognize the unrealistic position she'd been stuck in for her entire life. No wonder she was anxious all the time.

We spent several sessions clearing the old unresolved feelings with her father, since she had several memories that disturbed her. She was surprised to see that she had such strong feelings about her past and was amazed at how it had influenced her entire life. It was difficult for her to let go of her guilt for feeling these feelings, but over time it started to subside. It was clear from our work that she needed to heal the past in order to be more present with her son. At the end of her sessions involving her father, she was able to feel that she'd just been a child and that through no one's fault too much responsibility had been placed on her at a time when she just wanted to play and be a kid. As she dealt with the difficult feelings from her childhood, she came to accept that it was okay for her to feel unresolved and ambivalent emotions about her father and her childhood.

After completing her processing with her father, we continued to desensitize the present image of her son being late. Gradually, as she came to understand that she was taking on too much responsibility and trying to fix her unresolved emotional issues about her dad by trying to fix her son, her negative self-belief began to change. Once she processed the disturbance she felt, she began to accept the belief, "I'm a good mother," and we installed that belief until it had a VoC of 7. This was a huge relief to her. I had her let go of the images and look at any other triggers that might occur with her son. We worked on processing those pieces and then did mental future rehearsals of how she wanted to act and feel when interacting with her son.

Since then she has found it easier to let go and allow her son to be a normal teenager who must make his own mistakes and learn from them. By using EMDR, I was able to help Carolyn process her emotions in and through her body, achieve insight, and change her thoughts and behavior. She can now accept that her children are growing up and that she has done the best she could. By healing old, stuck places that created the traumatic symptom of anxiety, she has been able to shift enough emotionally so that her children don't stress her out as much and she feels less anxious, especially about her son. She's now able to recognize when a current situation is triggering something from her past and can choose her response rather than reacting out of old unresolved issues. Delving into her body as well as her mind, Carolyn has found a way to heal a traumatic experience in her childhood that was creating dysfunction in her present life.

Even though Carolyn's anxiety has lessened from the EMDR sessions concerning her interactions with her son, she continues to struggle with her anxiety and what makes her anxious and knows that there is more work to be done. Her commitment to her process is important and she continues to add more self-care to her routine. She recently decided to meditate on a daily basis. She's starting to track how her anxiety increases as the day goes on and is learning to make different choices along the way. She's realizing that her nervous system needs more retraining to achieve relaxation as a normal state. Her nervous system only needs to go on alert when needed to warn her of an actual danger. She's learning that to decrease her anxiety, she has to let go of the need to control that developed as a pattern in her childhood.

CHAPTER TEN

Overcoming Emotional Eating: Bob

Be that self which one truly is.

Soren Kierkegaard

Overeating is a common problem in the
United States. People suffering from weight issues are in the
news every day. We are bombarded with ads that tell us to
lose weight with whatever program is fast and easy. Unfortunately, one of the issues often overlooked is that eating may
have an emotional component. Many people who overeat may
be trying to control or soothe their feelings with food. Once
overweight, they begin to see their bodies as grotesque and
view themselves with hostility and contempt. They also hear
messages from the outside world that tell them they are fat
and, therefore, unlovable. When these voices become internalized, people learn to criticize themselves first even before others do. This critical voice becomes so powerful it feels as if it's
who they truly are. Sometimes the weight also creates a barrier
that keeps other people at a distance and that protects them
from things that they fear. When people feel isolated, lonely,
discouraged, and self-loathing, depression can become a way
of life.

Overeaters need to learn how to recognize when they are

competent in their world and giving toward others, and, especially, how to feel and tolerate their emotions. For many overweight people, eating and overeating has become a coping strategy for dealing with emotional pain. Not unlike alcohol or drugs, food can numb a painful feeling in the moment. Unfortunately, people often lose awareness and don't realize how much they have eaten. Along with the extra pounds, this sense of being out of control brings with it great shame. People will often hide what they are eating, eat when they're alone, and sometimes find shopping for groceries a painful experience. Also, unlike alcohol and drugs, food is everywhere, necessary for life, and a huge part of socialization, from family dinners to eating out. People whose eating is out of control are in a terrible bind. They have to eat to live. Their lives feel painful and out of control. Food soothes the pain for the moment but because their eating is out of control and adds weight, the end result is that they feel even more out of control and feel more pain. It's a vicious cycle in the form of a downward spiral that can end with severe health problems.

Learning to look at the issues underlying overeating and obesity is important to healing. For people who judge themselves harshly, it's important for them to remember that their disordered eating is how they survived whatever was happening in their life that was too painful to deal with. Food has been a substitute to fulfill real needs, such as to be seen, loved, and nurtured. Through years of repetition they have learned to eat without awareness and so have lost touch with the body's signals telling them that they are hungry or full.

Finding a safe environment in therapy to start expressing the distressing feelings that have been denied with food for so many years can be frightening. With EMDR clients can identify and work to heal the traumas that have contributed to overeating and obesity. Let's look at Bob's story about how he suffered from overeating and how EMDR helped him change his relationship to food.

Bob came into therapy seeking, he said, "deep change." He was a 47-year-old overweight architect who had spent years in talk therapy without seeing any results. He said that he had a lot of awareness of his issues but that awareness didn't seem to change anything. He had heard about EMDR through a friend and wanted to give it a try. Before I agreed, I needed to know more.

Bob presented himself as secure and strong in his body. He sat upright on the couch and held his breath ever so slightly. He was well dressed and showed a sense of confidence, but while he seemed in touch with his emotions as he talked, he felt embarrassed to tell me all about his life. With some encouragement, Bob admitted that he wasn't sleeping well, and he was overspending and overeating. He was trying to make a success of his business and often felt worthless. Underneath his social facade was an insecure, depressed man afraid to feel his feelings fully because there was just too much there that was painful and scary. When asked to describe how he looked inside, he came up with the image of a big black hole. If he let himself feel this, he said, he'd get lost in it and end up depressed for the rest of his life.

Bob's struggles with food were a huge concern for him. He had tried many diets and would lose weight and then gain it back with a little more, each time getting more and more frustrated. His history suggested a possible reason for his problem. Bob's mother had been thin and controlling with food. Bob had a big, strong body, but his mother labeled him overweight at an early age and put him on an endless and perpetual series of diets. He felt hungry all the time. As he watched his sisters eat whatever they wanted while his belly growled and his mouth watered, he felt deprived, alone, desperate, and needy. These feelings had continued into adulthood. Whenever he felt disturbing emotions—which was often—he turned to food. This left him feeling out of control, weak, ugly, and undesirable to women. I thought that if I could help Bob with these early memories about food, he might be able to gain a new perspective and make different and healthier choices now.

First we had to find a safe place for Bob. He chose his bedroom as an adult. He loved his room, the beautiful green color of the walls, and his special objects and his favorite books. He treasured his private space and loved thinking about it. As he contacted this feeling in his body, we added BLS with the pulsers. He loved the pulsers and looked forward to the sensations and how they helped reinforce his feeling of safety. We strengthened his safe place with the BLS until the feeling couldn't grow anymore.

For his container he imagined typing his feelings on his computer, downloading them to a file, transferring the file to a disk, erasing the file, and handing the disk to me. This step became an important piece of our work. Because so many things upset him in his life, he needed this coping skill to help him identify when he was upset versus when he was really hungry, as well as to find a way to contain the distressing feeling without resorting to food.

Next, I taught Bob deep belly breathing so that he would become aware when he was holding his breath. He tended to hold his breath often and not notice the effect it had on him—increased tension and anxiety.

As Bob worked through these exercises, he began to notice that he had more feelings than he ever imagined. He was also surprised that he often thought about food when he felt a distressing emotion. By learning to notice, identify, and then sit with an emotion, accepting it without trying to get rid of it too quickly, Bob improved his ability to listen to and reflect on his body's true signals.

After Bob had practiced his new skills at home and work, we decided that he was ready to do EMDR. Because he wanted to process with his eyes closed, he would open his eyes when he needed to stop. We then assessed his first target: his childhood memories of deprivation and humiliation.

- Image: "Watching everyone get a snack before dinner except me."
- Negative belief: "I'm unlovable because I'm fat."
- Positive belief: "I'm learning to feel good about myself the way I am."
- VoC scale: "2."
- Emotions: "Sadness, rage, and that life was unfair and I feel conflicted."
- SUDS scale: "9."
- Location of body sensation: "I feel a lump in my throat and coldness in my belly."

When we began the desensitization process, Bob's anger and resentment toward his mother burst forth. He felt hurt and enraged during the session, "sick" to his stomach with hate and frustration. Soon he came to a place where the process didn't seem to be working and he felt alone and afraid. While as a therapist I tend to trust the process, occasionally I find it necessary to step in. In EMDR, stepping in helps facilitate the process so that the client can proceed with the session. It's a way to help clients connect a truth that they already know with the reason why they're stuck, or to make it safe enough to continue. This was one of those times. I guided Bob to imagine who could come to help him with his feelings. He found a guardian angel that made it safe enough for him to continue his processing. When he brought his angel into the stuck scene, the process continued. He discovered that he believed comfort and approval came from someone outside of himself and that his inner guidance couldn't be trusted. He also couldn't trust his body-mind or read the signals it sent to let him know when he was really hungry or just seeking emotional comfort through food. The angel showed him that now that he was an adult, he was in charge of his choices; whenever he was upset or hungry his adult self could "feed" his inner child. Bob came to realize that he no longer needed to wait for outside permission or approval to attend to his own needs. This new ability gave him a sense of empowerment. He also began to feel compassion toward his mother; she wasn't a villain but had been trying to do a good thing with the diets out of fear for his health.

Bob needed three sessions to complete his work with this issue. By the end of the sessions, he felt that he was learning to feel that he was loveable and worthy of having his needs met—by himself. Since then he has developed a healthier relationship with his mother and a greater ability to listen to his own inner needs and feed his body with healthy food when he's hungry. He has also made a lifestyle change. He began working with a weight loss program that had him eat healthy foods. He lost the weight he wanted to lose and his positive sense of self increased enough that he wanted to start dating again. I helped him support these new, positive feelings with resource development installations whenever possible. Now when he slips and doesn't eat well, he understands that he was failed to listen to his own emotional needs. He's learning that his body communicates with his mind through how he eats, and that now, if he pays attention, he can make good choices. He has also realized that the black hole isn't quite as big after doing this work and has been willing to go deeper into it in search of more healing around other family issues.

CHAPTER ELEVEN

Moving Through Grief: Betsy

As soon as you trust yourself, you will know how to live.

Johann Wolfgang von Goethe

When you lose a loved one, the grief process has a natural rhythm. There is no right way to grieve and the experience is different for everyone. Grief has its own pace and timing and over time, when your processing system is working as it naturally does, you will move through your grief and gradually adjust to life without your loved one.

In normal grieving, from one minute to the next you may be flooded with memories of the good times or haunted by an image of a horrible ending that brings you tremendous pain and suffering. You may experience fatigue, insomnia, loss of appetite or overeating, anxiety, depression, and emotional numbness. Some people feel isolated and think that no one can understand what they are going through. Others may find themselves avoiding contact with other people out of fear that they may also leave, through death or desertion. You may experience conflicting feelings of relief that someone you care about is no longer in pain, and at the same time experience the pain of loss now that they're gone.

For some, grief may be experienced as a traumatic event.

When the processing system is interrupted and the loss can't be fully processed, it acts like a traumatic memory in your body-mind. This can create a sense of confusion and severely exacerbate and prolong grieving. At times you may not recognize what you are feeling as a symptom connected to traumatic grief. People often say to me, "Shouldn't I be over this already?" There is no timetable for your grief. You have to live your way through it.

If the grief seems especially severe in its impact on your life, or greatly prolonged, it may be that trauma is involved and you might want to seek out EMDR for help. When you lose a loved one, your world can change drastically and you may notice one or more of the following disruptions in your life:

- Questioning your basic beliefs about everything, especially life and death
- Confused thinking, difficulty concentrating, and memory problems
- Intense irritability or rage that is often misdirected
- General hopelessness, fear, frustration, and sadness
- A sense that everything feels out of control
- Physical complaints
- Lethargy
- Distressing dreams or intrusive images
- A strain in relationships
- Numbness
- A sense of detachment
- A sense of responsibility for the loss—feelings of guilt

EMDR has helped many people by relieving the symptoms of grief after a loss that hasn't been fully processed. Processing grief with EMDR does not mean that the grief will go away and that you won't feel the loss. Rather, it will support you while mourning the loss, help you let go of guilt or responsibility that does not belong to you, and allow you to remember the good memories that might earlier have been blocked. EMDR does not eliminate emotion but can help you accept the loss and find resolution in your own way. I've helped some people days after their loss, while others needed more time because they felt numb from head to toe and couldn't experience any feelings. Your therapist will help you assess if you are ready to do grief work with EMDR.

When you are grieving, it is important to take good care of yourself and be aware of the choices that you make. I let clients know that they need to be careful about watching too much news coverage because it is full of horrible death stories that can trigger loss. I recommend that you continue to reach out to other people and not isolate yourself. Sharing stories can help with the healing process and create a community of solidarity with others who have experienced loss, too. Eating well, avoiding alcohol, getting good rest, and exercising are a must, as is scaling back what you normally expect of yourself at home or at work. You just may not feel like you can do what you normally do.

Let's take a look at Betsy's story about losing her beloved dog, the pain she experienced, and how EMDR helped her come to some resolution with her loss.

Betsy was an attractive single woman of 32 who had for years been longing for a life partner. Professionally, she was a passionate holistic healer and loved helping people. Personally, however, she was insecure and turned to others for advice because she feared making mistakes. Often, she ended up making no decision at all. She lived with her dog, Toby, who was her closest companion, and dedicated hours to making sure he ate the right food, played outside in the woods, and in other ways got to spend "quality time" with her. Toby was her companion and best friend. She loved her time with Toby, and this relationship gave meaning to her life.

Toby was only 5 when he became ill and died unexpectedly. The shock of losing her companion was unbearable. Grief consumed Betsy's life. Everywhere she went, she was reminded of her beloved dog and her loss. She blamed herself for Toby's death because she'd discovered after the fact that she'd given him the wrong medication one time, a mistake she felt was unforgivable even though her dog had cancer. In her day-to-day life she struggled to do the simplest things and nothing gave her pleasure anymore due to her grief. While people were sympathetic, she knew that they also thought she was being overly dramatic, and sometimes she thought so, too. But no matter what she tried, she was unable to fill the void left by Toby's death. Her grief was affecting her work and relationships, but she didn't know what to do. Betsy's mother had heard of EMDR and thought it might help.

I agreed with Betsy's mom. Betsy was suffering from the trauma of the sudden, unexpected death of a beloved companion and held two negative self-beliefs, namely that she had been responsible for Toby's death and that she shouldn't be feeling what she was feeling. If she had been mourning a husband or a child, no one would question the validity of her grief, but for a dog? Clearly, they didn't understand and even Betsy questioned if she should feel this strongly for the loss of a pet. For Betsy, single, yearning for a partner and eventually for a child, Toby played an important role in her emotional life. The trauma of his loss was interfering with her ability to live.

As I got to know Betsy, she shared that she was having trouble concentrating and had lost interest in her work. She was often flooded with tears at unexpected times during the day and felt out of control. She'd lost her appetite and couldn't eat and whatever she ate went right through her. Betsy was a small, thin woman as it was and couldn't afford to lose any weight. She was haunted by the painful memories of the end of her dog's life journey, and recalling the decision she'd made to put him down was unbearable. Everywhere she looked, she saw Toby and what they'd done together. During our first conversation she was sobbing uncontrollably and the void she felt was palpable.

I told Betsy that while EMDR wouldn't stop the natural grieving process, I thought it could decrease her symptoms so that she could function at her job and feel more connected to people. When I asked about any other losses she'd suffered, she said there were none. That meant that we could focus on Toby's death.

We started by finding a safe place for Betsy because I wanted to help her feel more in control of her emotions. She remembered a time visiting Hawaii where she felt completely at home and at peace. I guided her to feel what it was like to lie on a warm beach and as she imagined her breath slowed and deepened and her body relaxed. We added BLS using hand tapping to reinforce the calm and peace she associated with her safe place, and to imprint these in her body-mind. Betsy did not like the other types of BLS and felt hand tapping was the most comfortable for her to experience. Her tears stopped flowing as she focused on her safe place and she felt thankful that she could stop crying.

For her container, Betsy imagined troubling emotions and issues filed away in my file cabinet. In her mind's eye she would see me lock them up so that she would not have to worry about them until I unlocked the cabinet at our next session.

Finally, I taught her belly breathing. I had her slow down, focus on her breath, and notice how it felt in her body. She reported that she could feel herself holding her breath and it was very hard to exhale. We started gently, just taking in a little inhale and then connecting the inhale with her exhale like a curve. Little by little as she focused and practiced, her breathing began to change. Eventually, she could take a full inhale and exhale. By the end of this session Betsy was feeling more in control of her breathing and her emotions.

Overall, Betsy's life was pretty stable. She had good friends, was close to her family, and knew she could get support if she ever needed it. She was successful at work and was in touch with her feelings. Her biggest issue, besides her grief, was her lack of confidence in herself and her decision making. This issue was definitely playing a part in her extreme grief. Doubting the choice she'd made to put her dog down still haunted her.

Once this preparatory work was complete, during our next session we turned to her traumatic event, Toby's death. Everything about it was painful to remember—"too painful," she at first insisted; she wasn't sure she was ready to go on. But after returning to her safe place and calming herself, she felt brave enough to follow my directions so that we could set up her stop signal—waving her hand ever so slightly—and then her first target of Toby's death. For Betsy, it turned out that there was no single worst image for her target. Each part of this traumatic event was a SUDS 10 and had to be worked on piece by piece, creating several targets. We began at the beginning.

- Image: "Poor Toby, sick and barely able to move."
- Negative belief: "It's all my fault. I'm a bad person."
- Positive belief: "It wasn't my fault and I'm a good person. I loved him as much as I could."
- VoC scale: "2."
- Emotions: "Sorrow, anger at myself and Toby's vet, and guilt!"
- SUDS scale: "10."
- Location of body sensation: "I feel sensations in my heart and throat."

I began the desensitization BLS using hand tapping. She used very long sets, riding the emotional waves as if she was surfing her traumatic experience. Each scene of the event would appear as if she were in a movie. She reported that each piece was just as painful as the next: noticing that Toby was ill; getting him to the hospital; seeing him in pain; finding out about the wrong medication; the veterinarian saying that there was no hope; her feeling helpless and alone; Toby dying in her arms; seeing places that reminded her of Toby after he was gone. After this first session, some of the scenes were down to a SUDS 0, but some of the later parts that she hadn't gotten to yet still felt high in disturbance. She had a distance to go to finish this work.

Her sessions were very emotional and she would often sob for minutes at a time. The pain was difficult for her to bear but after each time she cried, she reported feeling better. She didn't have to share many of the details for the processing to work. My job was to keep her processing moving forward. After almost every session, her SUDS score was 0 for the target we were working on that day. When occasionally she still felt disturbed at the end of a session, she filed the disturbing parts away in my filing cabinet and in her mind's eye I locked the drawer.

Betsy's EMDR took several weeks to complete. With each session she untangled a bit more of the self-blame that had been torturing her. Gradually, she came to realize that she hadn't caused Toby's death. His dying was beyond her control. Over time, she developed a sense of compassion and forgiveness for herself. Her new positive belief turned into "I loved him as much as I could, and always do the best I can." Through the weeks we worked together, she started exploring what to do in the free time that Toby's absence had opened up for her. Instead of asking friends, she began to ask herself what kinds of things she'd like to do and started reaching out to people and, when opportunities arose, taking some chances. Her appetite slowly returned: her concentration improved; and she challenged herself with new projects at work to keep her interest piqued. Her nightmares ended and she felt stronger and more confident in her life.

After her EMDR therapy was complete on this issue, we decided to work on other issues—her yearning for a partner and her troubles at work. Betsy started school to prepare for her pursuit of a new career, made new friends, and even started dating. She recalls Toby with love, and says she will never forget the experience of his death. But now, when she remembers, it's a quiet recollection without the symptoms of trauma that had threatened her job, her relationships, and her sense of self. Although Betsy would rather that Toby had lived, in a way, she's now as grateful for his death as she always was for his love. Toby's dying, even the way he died, turned out to be what writer C. S. Lewis once called a "severe mercy": Toby's final gift to Betsy was to compel her through grief to seek therapy and, with the help of EMDR, to learn to live her life in a new and fuller way.

When the one-year anniversary of Toby's death approached, some of Betsy's guilt returned. She began to question her decisions again. We again used EMDR to help her sort out the truth and come to some resolution. I took her through the pieces that felt stuck and had for some reason not fully come to resolution in our first sessions. She realized that she was fearful that others could die in the future and she would be all alone.

Grief can be triggered by anniversaries and if symptoms arise, that is okay, normal, and natural. Betsy's loss has made her question what she believes about life and death, the difficult choices as adults we sometimes have to make, and learn that she can handle whatever comes up in her life. She bravely faces her experiences and welcomes whatever she can learn about herself and life through EMDR. Her journey is a path that she is fully committed to and when she struggles, she comes in for sessions to help her find her inner strength and truth. Her EMDR experience has helped her move through her grief one step at a time at her own pace.

CHAPTER TWELVE

Finding Courage After Sexual Abuse: Joan

In the middle of difficulty lies opportunity.

Albert Einstein

Sexual abuse is common in our culture, but it is not an easy subject to discuss. One out of every three girls is sexually abused in childhood, and one out of every seven boys. That is an alarming statistic and probably underreported. The effects of sexual abuse are often devastating. With abuse there is a power differential that factors into the pain. The perpetrator has the power and the victim tends to become passive or submissive in order to survive the abuse. The boundary violation is confusing for victims and they are left feeling powerless to change the situation. As the perpetrator manipulates to control, the victim tries to find ways to survive and not feel pain, such as holding her breath or freezing. Some victims dissociate from the pain and even experience themselves leaving their bodies to escape. Often, victims end up feeling invisible and as if they don't matter. Sexual abuse can create a huge hole that will block people's energy, their life force, their sexuality, and their ability to be emotionally intimate later in life.

Over the years I have seen many women who have been sexually abused at some point in their life. They have always known their perpetrator and struggle with this knowledge. Sometimes they're in denial. Their emotions range from numbness to hypersensitivity. They may feel shame or disgust at another's touch, avoid certain places, or seek out inappropriate attention. They often experience fear, panic, depression, substance abuse, suicidal and intrusive thoughts, recurring nightmares, health issues, eating disorders, and relationship problems. Fortunately, EMDR can help.

Joan came in for therapy because she felt like she was falling apart and knew she needed professional help. She was a single woman, age 25, studying for her master's degree. Her life seemed to be manageable until she started school again. Now she was feeling completely overwhelmed and struggling in her psychology classes because they were triggering an earlier event in her life. Even before a class would begin, her heart would start racing, she could hardly breathe, and all she wanted to do was run. She felt anxious all the time, never safe, and rarely comfortable, and spent a lot of time hiding this from everyone she knew. It was difficult to socialize because everyone else seemed to have it all together and she couldn't let on to her classmates that she was falling apart. To relieve anxiety, Joan found herself self-medicating with alcohol and feared developing alcoholism. After spending almost 3 years in more traditional psychotherapy, she had a thorough awareness of her issues and thought that she was ready for a more integrative approach. She said, "I've talked and talked and talked around my traumas for years," but she still felt very damaged and was struggling to function in her daily life. Now she wanted to actually move the trauma through and out of her body.

In gathering her history, I learned that during her senior year in high school Joan had had a year-long affair with one of her teachers. She'd felt so much shame from the affair that she became depressed and shut down emotionally. She said, "The spark went out of me and I vanished inside." Although she'd been a good student, she lost her internal compass and it took everything she had to hold herself together, graduate, and go on to college. There she discovered that her relationships with men had been fatally compromised. Each relationship became a replay of her traumatic affair. To forget the pain of this, she began to party. She sexualized friendships, didn't know how to be in the company of men without seeing herself as a sexual object, and had sex before she felt ready for that degree of intimacy. Once in a relationship she reacted as if her boyfriend was trying to smother her and take away her autonomy, and what intimacy they shared soon disintegrated into screaming, crying, and accusations. Men: she couldn't trust any of them. But without them she felt lonely and lost, and to numb her pain she drank more alcohol. She felt that there was something in her body that shouldn't be there, that she was dirty, and despite her intelligence, education, and years of therapy, she didn't know how to get rid of these sensations, emotions, and thoughts. All this and she was only in her mid-20s.

Clearly, Joan was being triggered repeatedly by studying and talking about trauma in her psychology class. This was activating her own trauma response. She felt tremendous pressure to be a good student, but studying to be a therapist was proving more challenging than she'd expected. A passionate woman with a huge heart, she longed to help people. Before she could do so, however, she had to find a way to deal with her own trauma, which was evoked continually in the context of lectures and the experiential work that students were required to do on their own issues. Repeatedly, her amygdala was triggered by statements she heard in class, or by self-reflection, or by a male teacher she respected but feared.

As Joan entered my office, she was so fearful that nothing could help her that her body was shaking, and I knew that I had to quickly help her find a way to calm her nervous system and regain her confidence. Her fear of feeling out of control kept her in a state of panic and distrust. I immediately taught her a grounding exercise. I asked her to imagine that she was a strong tree feeling her roots holding her upright, supporting her trunk—her body's torso. This helped calm her down in the office, and when she began to practice at home she found that when she connected to this imagery and felt it in her body-mind, it evoked a sense of inner strength. I also taught her belly breathing in order to slow down and calm her nervous system. Joan loved the tree meditation and felt instant relief.

Next, she needed to find her safe place. It was on a beach she had once visited. Joan was an avid yogi but had stopped her yoga practice once she started school. We needed to get those skills back to support her process. I invited her to remember her deep belly breathing from yoga, to slow down and ask all of her to be at the beach. Once she managed this, a huge grin appeared on her face, her body tension released, and she sank into the couch. I reinforced this with BLS. She loved the pulsers and earphones used together, which was somehow soothing to her, and she couldn't wait to visit her safe place on the beach.

Her container was a bit different. She put disturbing thoughts, emotions, and issues away by taking a deep breath, feeling her feet on the ground, focusing on her current environment—shapes, colors, sounds, textures, objects—and then relaxing, letting the tension and thoughts go. I sent Joan home to practice these skills—safe place, containment, and deep breathing. She also decided that she needed to start up her yoga practice again because she realized that she really missed it. I was happy for her to reengage in something that was good for her and could help diminish her trauma activation.

As Joan's awareness increased, she noticed what specifically triggered her at school. I kept notes of these triggers. In general, it was her trauma therapy class, her sexuality class, and the way her male teacher talked to her. She started practicing her resourcing in class. When she felt the first sign of activation, in her mind's eye she would go to her safe place. She started feeling stronger and more confident as time went by.

As we talked, I learned more about her family history and what it was like growing up in her household. She'd been a vibrant young girl, with an older sister who needed a lot of attention. Her mother suffered from cancer but survived and her sister struggled with schizophrenia, which was very hard on the whole family. Joan was worried about losing her mother and how to relate to her sister, constantly feeling abandoned by her family. She made some very close friends in school, but one day the group abandoned her, leaving her alone and fearful. Who was there to care for her and comfort her? Where was her support? From this place of need, a teacher saw and took advantage of a girl in desperate need of attention and love.

Joan knew this abusive relationship was the beginning of so many of the symptoms wreaking havoc on her ability to sustain a healthy, intimate relationship with a man. As an intelligent graduate student, she'd understood for a long time that her teacher had abused his power over a teenage girl flattered by his attention and that it was he who should have been responsible for setting boundaries. The adult part of her knew that this was an abuse of power, but her child part felt it was a love affair. She couldn't reconcile the two. As she explored the traumatic experience, she began to feel in her body what she'd felt when she'd started to stay after class to talk to him because he was friendly and kind and listened sympathetically about her struggles in school. He lavished her with attention and compliments and eventually initiated the sexual relationship. She felt flattered and deeply ambivalent. She felt that she couldn't refuse but once it happened, although she felt some pleasure, most of the time she felt internal confusion. She needed to be loved and cared for and he was providing that, so she thought. It was only later that she realized that he had taken advantage of her and manipulated her so that she became dependent on him. Through her previous talk therapy she'd come to understand that no matter how much he professed to care about her, he had used his authority and power to sexually abuse her. But this was an intellectual understanding she did not feel in her body. Even though she knew better, she still blamed herself. After all, she'd been a willing participant; didn't that mean that she was responsible? Now, in college, when Joan felt alone and powerless, unable to feel safe or connect with men, and fearful that she would never again make good choices, she found herself haunted by self-loathing.

Like many victims of abuse, part of Joan believed that she somehow had caused the abuse. Indeed, perpetrators often reinforce this belief in order to shift responsibility and assuage their own guilt. The lack of safety in the relationship is also confusing because the victim is encouraged by the perpetrator to keep their secret in order to protect him and their relationship. However, with her intellectual understanding about what happened, it was time for Joan to move the stuck feelings out of her body and mind.

She chose her stop signal. We assessed as the target the sexual relationship she had with her teacher in high school.

- Image: "The horrible grimace on his face when he's having sex with me."
- Negative belief: "I'm disgusting and helpless."
- Positive belief: "Now is different than then; I'm strong and lovable."
- VoC scale: "2."
- Emotions: "Despair, despondent, dead."
- SUDS scale: "10."
- Location of body sensation: "Sensations in my chest and heart."

Joan used the pulsers and earphones for her BLS and her sessions were intense. There were times when she thought she couldn't do the desensitization, but she always managed to find the courage deep within to face this teacher once again, knowing that now was different than then. She trembled and cried and sometimes needed support from an internal team of guides whenever she felt stuck in the process—in her mind, her internal team consisted of actual new friends from college who didn't judge her and accepted her for who she really was. She imagined that these friends would provide safety so that she could look at the past and know she was safe in the present.

After the first session, it was clear that her work was not complete and I had her contain the rest of the disturbance for a later date. We ended each session with her going to her safe place and finding relaxation. She came in the next week noting that for two days she'd been extremely exhausted from our last session but that she was doing okay in school. She felt ready to complete this nightmare, so we finished the memory of the abuse in this next session. During the desensitization she felt sadness, fear, and pain, and she often cried, especially as she became increasingly aware in her body of her inability to establish clear boundaries and how this affected her ability to relate to men. She began to understand at a physical level what she'd previously grasped intellectually; that the abuse had permeated her relationships and made it difficult to trust or have an intimate relationship with a man when she feared the power that men seemed to have over her. But by the end of the session Joan was able to bring the image of the teacher to mind without any emotional activation in her body. She easily moved into the belief, "I'm strong and lovable," and we installed it. She said the feeling was growing and growing and she didn't want it to stop. I let her continue the sets of installation until she felt it was as strong a feeling as it could be.

To make sure we had cleared this entire piece, I asked Joan to be aware of any current triggers in her life. She told me she had a mandatory meeting with her feared male professor. She dreaded this meeting and felt anxious. She anticipated that the meeting would provoke now-conscious fear that a teacher with power would hurt her again. We cleared this trigger with EMDR desensitization and did an installation until she felt ready and prepared to face this teacher.

At our next session, she reported that the meeting had gone well with her teacher. She'd had no physical reaction when she saw him. She was able to speak to him clearly, and realized with astonishment that she was a different person. She'd forgotten how life felt without fear. She'd given up the hope that she could interact with a man, any man, without wariness and caution. EMDR changed this forever. Our work on this was done for now. With the help of EMDR, Joan's healing had reached the level of her body-mind. The traumatic memories and emotions that had been fragmented and stored were now released and resolved. The abuse was in the past where it belonged.

As therapy progressed Joan felt stronger and more confident and the realization that it's okay to say no to a man moved from her intellect into her body-mind. As she expressed anger and rage in therapy at the teacher who'd abused her, she found compassion for herself and her self-blame gradually dissipated. She still drank occasionally but no longer self-medicated with alcohol. Tentatively at first, she began exploring a relationship with a man who made it safe for her to set boundaries, to be vulnerable and tell the truth, and to say no whenever she felt the need.

By having the courage to face a huge fear and trusting the EMDR process, Joan's life changed dramatically. She continued in therapy to deal with some other issues in her childhood that have also caused her distress.

CHAPTER THIRTEEN

Defeating the Devastation of War: Sam

You gain strength, courage, and confidence by every experience in which you really stop to look fear in the face. You are able to say to yourself, I have lived through this horror. I can take the next thing that comes along. You must do the thing you think you cannot do.

Eleanor Roosevelt

As I mentioned earlier in the book, Francine Shapiro developed EMDR by working with people who suffered from PTSD. Her first PTSD research study included U.S. veterans damaged emotionally in the Vietnam War. Let's look more closely at a Vietnam vet who finally sought treatment with EMDR.

Sam joined the army back in the early 1970s and with his college education was sent to officer training school. Despite basic training, when he got to Vietnam he was not prepared for the sudden onset or intensity of battle. Just after he arrived, as he was leading his unit along a road at night, the enemy suddenly opened up with mortar and machine-gun fire. The unseasoned troops panicked, and many were killed. During Sam's 2-year tour in Vietnam, there were many other combat situations in which the enemy was unseen until the moment he and his troops were attacked. There were also many times that he led his troops into villages to fight and kill enemy guerillas who afterward turned out to be women and children.

When he returned to the United States and resigned from the army, Sam suffered from recurring nightmares and found that he was unable to get along with his bosses on the job. He would react to demands at work by either walking away or getting into angry arguments. Over the years he lost a number of jobs, moving down through demotions from professional manager to operations supervisor to eventually working on an assembly line. Because of his moodiness, his impatience, and his drinking, his marriage fell apart soon after his return to the States. He had several relationships, none of which lasted more than 2 years. He became dependent on alcohol, and his social circle consisted of his buddies in the bar.

Sam finally came for therapy 30 years after he'd left Vietnam. A friend who had been successfully treated with EMDR for her panic disorder referred him for treatment. She feared for his health, and his occasional statements that life was not worth living made her worry about suicide.

By the time Sam started counseling, he was sharing a mobile home in a trailer park and saw himself as a failure with little to live for. He presented with all the classic signs of PTSD. He felt stressed all the time. He couldn't assert or stand up for himself. He felt anxious and depressed and dreaded going to work out of fear of negative interactions with people as a result of his angry outbursts. He drank heavily in order to numb emotional pain, and yet the alcohol just made things worse. Any loud noise startled him. His nightmares were getting more frequent and disturbing. He looked worn out, with dark circles under his eyes. His jaw was tightly clenched and his body rigid. He clearly had no internal resources and very few external resources to help him feel stable and secure in his life.

Sam began therapy by telling his stories from the war. This appeared challenging for him; he seemed to be testing the counseling process to see if he would be judged as incompetent or a bad person. As he revealed more about his history, his internal resources were being developed and strengthened.

First, Sam had to learn how to deep belly breathe to slow down his nervous system and relieve himself of his constant need to remain on guard. He also practiced how to feel and recognize his emotions without the need to change or push them away. He slowly learned to track the sensations in his body without judgment, knowing he was safe in this moment in time. He worked on understanding that "here and now" in the office was not "there and then" in the war.

Sam also needed to deal with his drinking so that alcohol would not exacerbate his symptoms or impede the therapy. He agreed to start Alcoholics Anonymous and to stay away from bars. In addition to teaching him how alcohol was sabotaging his efforts to find meaning in his life, AA also helped him increase his external network of people. He also agreed to start sharing what he felt with a good friend.

Through the resource development phase, Sam found his own safe place in the image of a riverside camp in the high mountains. For a container he pictured a tightly tied duffel bag put in a storage shed that was locked with three padlocks.

At the same time, Sam was told about EMDR and how it works, and that until the trauma was fully processed there could be times when he might feel increased agitation and have nightmares as a part of the processing. He agreed that he was now ready to face the past that was haunting him.

Finding EMDR targets for Sam was complicated, since there were so many horrific images and upsetting events from his Vietnam days and often the memories were blended together. To help make it safer for him, a modification to the normal EMDR approach was used. Instead of focusing on individual images, his stories were processed by putting them into a form of home movie. Sam was the screenwriter, director, and photographer. He could show them on his mental movie screen and run the movie at the speed that worked for him, holding the imaginary controls in his hands to stop and start whenever he needed. Here is the beginning assessment of his target, which was a starting place for the work.

- Image: "The night my platoon was attacked on the road and the flashes of light from the explosions and the sounds of the wounded soldiers crying out."
- Negative belief: "I'm incompetent."
- Positive belief: "I'm capable."
- VoC scale: "2."
- Emotions: "Fear, anger, guilt, anxiety."
- SUDS scale: "9."
- Location of body sensation: "In my stomach and then up to my neck."

Sam used eye movements for the BLS during the desensitization phase. He would start with the picture of an event and then let the video sequence play without having to describe any of the details. During the sets Sam would twitch throughout his entire body while tears rolled down his face. He had observable periods of silence while he was revisiting an event in his memory. As he processed each target it seemed difficult to reduce the SUDS level because another event immediately following in the "video" remained unresolved. However, after four EMDR sessions the disturbance he felt had lowered considerably. His nightmares diminished and his flashbacks were less frequent and milder. He also began to remember additional memories that he had forgotten.

The next target was set up the same way. He now understood and accepted that he might not be able to fully process each target completely in the session, since there were so many pieces to this horrific experience. He continued for several sessions, working piece by piece, until he felt relief of his symptoms.

In the last session, Sam was asked to review the entire movie in his mind again, making sure to notice any disturbance. At this point in the desensitization with the BLS, a particularly strong memory came back to him. He remembered getting separated from his platoon and walking into an ambush. He was captured, tied to a tree, stuck with a bayonet, and left to die. The next thing he remembered was waking up in a field hospital. His immediate and lasting reaction to this event was that he had been incompetent and failed his troops by letting himself be captured. This memory came as a complete surprise to him and needed to be cleared. As he processed it, the disturbance increased and then completely disappeared by the end of the session.

Sam was able to calmly review the movie without feeling anything that disturbed him after all the key targets were processed. He moved naturally into the belief "I'm capable" and felt it in his body, mind, and soul. The installation of his belief with the entire movie was reinforced and integrated.

The next step was to look at any current triggers in his life that might need work with EMDR. He didn't find any current triggers but wanted to work on future issues to support his feeling of "I'm capable." This included preparing for a new job.

After Sam completed these sessions, he found the courage to leave the assembly line and he found a more professional job. A year later he applied for and won a manager's position. He stopped drinking and saved his money to move into an apartment. Sam is appreciative of the new life he has created with the help of EMDR, and now promotes the treatment to other vets so that they, too, can get help with their war-caused emotional pain.

CHAPTER FOURTEEN

Reclaiming Power After Rape: Rebecca

Patience and perseverance have a magical effect before which difficulties disappear and obstacles vanish.

John Quincy Adams

"No" really does mean "no." No one has the right to have sex with you without your consent. What you wear, what you say, or how you act never justifies rape. The blame for any rape lies solely with the rapist. Anyone can be raped, female or male. Gender and age are not a factor.

When a person is raped, his or her world turns upside down. The act of rape isn't just about sex—it's about power over another human being. There is no typical rapist. Rape can happen with a stranger, a date, an acquaintance, or even a family member. But no matter how or with whom it happens, victims may be left feeling frightened and traumatized. Their world no longer feels safe and it's harder for them to trust people. What happens after a rape is also often difficult and can be just as harmful to the victim as the rape itself. Many victims choose not to report rapes to the police because they feel ashamed of what happened, and the tendency to blame themselves is all too often reinforced by skeptical, unsympathetic police officers, although this is changing. What happens after a rape can lessen or worsen the effects of the actual trauma of the rape. When the victim tells someone, is she believed? What kind of support does she receive? What was her treatment by the police? How do her family and friends react? Is she offered medical treatment? Each part of this event can be harmful if the victim does not feel supported and responded to in an empathetic manner.

If you are raped, it is important to seek medical care as soon as possible. Most hospitals have emergency care with doctors and counselors who have been trained to help. The doctor will need to check you for sexually transmitted diseases, internal injuries, and any evidence of the crime. Most towns and cities also have rape hotlines and crisis centers that you can call for advice from advocates who can go with you and help you through this process. Experts suggest that you do not change your clothes, shower, douche, or wash after a rape until after you have been checked medically. Of course, you want to clean up, but you need to get the right medical care immediately and if you choose to report the crime you will need physical evidence. Even if you don't report it right away, should you decide to do so later, it's important that the evidence be available.

Rape is a big-T trauma, one of the most traumatic events a person can suffer outside of combat. In a way, it is combat, but with a strong and sneaky foe. After a rape you may feel angry, degraded, frightened, numb, confused, ashamed and embarrassed, depressed, anxious, nervous, and alone. You may experience symptoms of PTSD such as difficulty sleeping, loss of appetite, difficulty concentrating, nightmares, and intrusive images. Some women withdraw from the support of family and friends out of fear that they're being judged. It is important for you to seek out professional guidance in an environment that feels safe in order to get the help you need.

Here is a story that illustrates how a traumatic event devastated a woman's life and how EMDR helped her reclaim her power.

Rebecca was single and 31 when she came into therapy. She'd been raped a year before and was feeling increasingly anxious and depressed. She was a tall, lean, beautiful woman who looked incredibly frail. As she sat on my couch, I wondered how she managed to get through her day. She spoke very softly, was extremely nervous, almost shaking, and reminded me of a wounded bird with whom I'd have to be very gentle.

She said that she felt like she'd been in shock since the rape and worried about how her traumatic symptoms were affecting everyone around her. She wasn't taking care of herself, felt overwhelmed by even the smallest responsibilities and often thought she was going crazy. She knew who had attacked her and could not let go of what she suspected was a futile effort to collect evidence and have her attacker arrested and punished. By constantly obsessing about whether people believed her story and thinking how she could punish the rapist, she was making herself and everyone around her miserable.

I gathered enough of her history to know that she'd had a difficult childhood. Her parents separated when she was 2 and from then on she lived with her mother and her older half brother and half sister. Her mother, an alcoholic and drug addict, would often leave the children home alone. They moved frequently, and these moves made Rebecca feel insecure. She felt jumpy around her mother and brother and learned to keep quiet and stay out of their way. She said that she now felt the same with her boyfriend. Her mother attempted suicide three times and physically assaulted Rebecca's sister, brother, and sometimes even strangers. Her brother molested her when she was 6 and she was afraid to tell anyone.

When she was 7 her father remarried and got custody of the children, and from then on life was pretty stable. Still, she described her childhood as a black hole and hated to think about it. As an adult, her sister became a heroin addict. Rebecca no longer spoke to her brother. Her relationship with her mother had healed somewhat and she now felt closer to her than to the rest of her family.

Although Rebecca's history was full of trauma, she functioned pretty well until the rape. Since then she'd tried a couple of talk therapy sessions to deal with her traumatic symptoms but felt she couldn't trust her male therapist. In fact, even though I was a woman, she believed that she was taking a huge risk coming to see me. More or less successfully, Rebecca had spent a lot of time and energy through the years attempting to forget her history of childhood trauma. She seldom spoke up, stayed out of the way, and walked on eggshells. The rape made this suppression impossible. I could see that it was going to be hard for her to trust me or for her to believe that EMDR could help.

It was obvious that Rebecca lived in a constant state of hyperarousal. When I made this observation, she agreed. She said that she knew she was unreasonably hypervigilant; she felt on guard with everyone, couldn't trust anyone, and would jump at the slightest noise. She had difficulty concentrating and making decisions, and found herself irritable, angry, and depressed most of the time. She had night sweats and recurring nightmares and flashbacks about the rape. During the day, without any warning, she would find herself reliving some aspect of the rape. She wanted to be sexual but was struggling sexually with her boyfriend. She described herself as in survival mode and wouldn't make any long-term plans or goals out of fear of what could happen in the future. She was afraid to remember the trauma but knew she couldn't get on with her life until she'd dealt with the rape. Clearly, Rebecca was suffering all the classic symptoms of PTSD.

Rebecca had reacted to the rape by freezing, but in an involuntary and unusual manner. The rape had happened at her cousin's wedding. "You think you can trust people at a wedding," she said, and so her guard was down. She'd been drinking alcohol and, a bit tipsy, she and a man she'd met began to "have fun." She remembered little after that. Had she been drugged? This was all Rebecca could tell me in our first session. She was too embarrassed to tell me everything that had occurred and I did not pressure her for details. From the magnitude of her PTSD symptoms it was clear that something else had happened to her, but there was no need to press. I knew that through the EMDR process more details would emerge as Rebecca felt safer. One beauty of EMDR is that, as a therapist, I don't need to know all the details for the therapy to work.

What she remembered and was able to talk about was waking up naked in a hotel room, sore, bruised, and not knowing what had happened or what to do. Her body hurt but her mind was blank. Her father found her and she went with him to her home state, where she went to a hospital. Unfortunately, by then it was too late to test for a date rape drug or DNA. When a male detective came to see her, he accused her of making up the story to ruin the accused man's life. She felt devalued and betrayed. This experience further traumatized her and exacerbated her chronic self-doubt. Fortunately, more and more hospitals are educating their staff on proper treatment for rape victims so that people don't have to experience what Rebecca did in this case.

Although she couldn't remember the actual rape, she was haunted by nightmares and flashbacks and her mind kept futilely trying to fill in the empty places in her memory in order to make some sense of the horror.

Clearly, Rebecca had suffered a big-T trauma. Although she couldn't remember the actual event, from the state of her body when she came to, it was apparent that the rape had been rough, if not violent, and Rebecca felt overwhelmed by what she could remember and what she could not. Despite the absence of conscious memory, her body-mind knew what had happened and she was flooded by images, emotions, and physical sensations, including sounds and smells. Rebecca desperately wanted to trust her experience, but the constant stress-induced neurochemical cascade in her brain and body continually disrupted her ability to process information about the rape. She thought if she just tried harder to remember the rape, then she would be okay. Trying to remember was causing her to obsess about what had happened. Unable to fill in the blanks, yet tormented by nightmares and intrusive thoughts and sensations, Rebecca's self-doubt increased, and this was exacerbating her symptoms.

Because she had suffered earlier traumas as a child, the rape had also activated many associated traumatic memories that for years she'd been able to suppress. From her childhood experience, Rebecca had developed the personality of a cautious woman who did her best to fly under the radar and never make waves. Her major defense mechanism seemed to be denial, which had now broken down completely. Although she was currently living with her boyfriend, she doubted his ability to support her because she felt betrayed by his doubt about the rape. When she finally came to see me, what support system she had was shaky and built on an unstable childhood foundation. All this made her more vulnerable; she just couldn't trust people and felt that she had to keep it all together herself, something that now she couldn't do.

My first task was to help Rebecca develop some inner resources and feel more stable in her life. We began our work by finding a safe place. I did not use the term "safe place" with Rebecca because she wasn't feeling safe in her world. I instead asked her to find a peaceful place. Rebecca found relief and safety in the image of a frozen lake with snow-covered hills where everything was white, calm, and refreshing. For the first time in years her body softened, her breathing eased, and her overactive sympathetic nervous system calmed down. As she calmed her nervous system, I added BLS using eye movement to strengthen and support this new feeling state.

Next, we found a container. She chose a big canvas bag. I asked her if she really felt like she could contain any disturbance in the bag. After some reflection, she said, "No, I need to tie a big rope around it and then put it in a large trunk." Still uncertain if this would be strong enough for her, I asked again if this felt right, and again she said, "No, I need to lock the trunk and put it in a concrete basement." Once she had this image, I asked her to think of a little upset from the week. She remembered a fight with her boyfriend that clearly still agitated her. I asked her to put the fight in her container and seal it up good and tight. She did this. Then I asked her to return in her mind's eye to her peaceful place. Again, her breathing slowed and her sympathetic nervous system calmed down.

I then explained the importance of breath in the process of healing. I asked her to notice how she was breathing. She was breathing shallowly and often held her breath, like a frightened animal trying to disappear. I had her put both hands on her abdomen and imagine a balloon inside her belly; when she inhaled, she filled the balloon with air, and when she exhaled all the air flowed out of the balloon through her mouth. This took some practice, but once she slowed down her breathing she began to feel the difference in her body. She practiced this work at home and reported at each session that she was feeling better and was relieved that something was helping her. Now that she was able to calm her nervous system and relax her body, I knew that we were ready to move into EMDR sessions.

Before we started EMDR desensitization, it was difficult for Rebecca to remember or talk about the rape. What memories she had were painful and she was afraid to feel them. I assured her that she did not need to tell me anything she wasn't ready to tell. I didn't need a lot of details—this was for her to experience, not for me to know. We assessed the target of her being raped since this was the most dominant memory that was interrupting her life.

- Image: "Seeing my father's face when he found me naked on the hotel bed."
- Negative belief: "I'm disgusting."
- Positive belief: "I did nothing wrong. I'm okay."
- VoC scale: "2."
- Emotions: "Fear, confusion."
- SUDS scale: "10."
- Location of body sensation: "Hips, legs, jaw."

Rebecca used eye movement for her processing with BLS and said she would close her eyes if she needed to stop for some reason. As she began to trust the process, she moved through her fear with courage. She allowed herself to feel anger that she had previously not been able to express. The sessions were not as difficult as Rebecca feared and she was amazed that she could do the EMDR and feel change every week.

It took five sessions to move through the experience of the rape step by step, image by image, sensation by sensation, emotion by emotion, as she processed the horror and began to integrate the memories of what had happened to her. The fifth session was the hardest for her to finish. She was still haunted by not knowing what had truly taken place. I asked her to imagine what she thought had happened, seeing all the details and feeling free to make it up as she went along as if it were a dream. By giving her permission to imagine what had happened, she was able to process this part of the horror. The purpose was not to retrieve a memory, but rather to give her permission to feel what she was so afraid to feel. This allowed her to process the memory whether it was the literal truth or not. Her brain wanted to fill in the blanks to make sense of what she felt. She never told me what she envisioned, but the results were clear. She was free from her nightmares. Once the trauma fully processed, she was now able to feel her positive belief, "I did nothing wrong, I'm okay." She was able to integrate this new belief fully into the memory and begin to explore this in the rest of her life.

When we fully completed this target, Rebecca noticed some changes that she reported in her next session. She began to sleep better and her nightmares disappeared. She started to reclaim some personal power and a sense that she could assert herself. She started setting boundaries with people by saying "no." She realized that her relationship with an unsupportive man was unhealthy and decided to leave him so that she could focus on taking better care of herself. She no longer felt obsessed with her attacker or thought that she was going crazy. She let go of needing to know exactly what had happened to her and no longer felt compelled to prosecute her attacker. She just wanted to get on with her life. As her internal strength grew, she felt safer in the world. She still remembered the rape, but the PTSD symptoms disappeared. Rebecca came into my office looking like a new woman who had reclaimed her power on an internal level, and this was now reflected in her body and mind. She stood straighter and seemed more solid. Her voice was stronger. She was proud of the new choices she was now making in her life. On the 2-year anniversary of the rape she reported that while she still remembered, no part of it haunted her anymore. She remained a bit surprised but very grateful that she no longer had to live stuck in that past horror.

After we completed EMDR work on the rape, we went back into her childhood to resolve a number of disturbing traumas, especially her mother's instability and the molestation by her brother. Over time Rebecca continued to grow stronger and more confident, found a new job, and planned to go back to school. Slowly, she is overcoming a childhood of emotional deprivation and fear, learning how to assert herself, and finding the courage to do so. Today, mostly recovered from her traumas, life is fuller than it's ever been and she's living in ways that bring her more joy.

CHAPTER FIFTEEN

Conquering Fear: Tyler and Robert

Do the thing we fear, and death of fear is certain.

Ralph Waldo Emerson

In EMDR terms, there are two classifications of phobias: simple and process. A simple phobia is a fear of something specific such as spiders, dogs, or snakes. The fear occurs from actually seeing something, which activates a fear response and a cascade of sensations in the body. A process phobia is more complicated. A person will be in a complex situation that triggers fear repeatedly throughout the experience. The most common example is flying. There are many aspects to a process phobia. With flying, for example, you have to figure out when to fly, buy the tickets, find a way to the airport, check your bags, hear terrorist security warnings, pass through security, wait for the plane, and then get on the plane. Then the plane must take off and land and you have to get to your final destination.

With EMDR, the simple phobia is much easier to treat than the process phobia. The simple phobia is targeted with one image, usually imaginary. With a process phobia the client has to work with each piece of the process that contributes to the phobia until the whole thing is integrated. In both cases, the person needs help to learn how to handle fear of fear. I always take a history to determine the first time the fear occurred, the most disturbing aspect of the phobia, and the most recent occurrence if there is one. Once that's done, we target current triggers.

Simple Phobia: Tyler

Tyler was a 26-year-old man who was physically strong and fit. He had a professional job and was married. He came into therapy specifically because of his fear of spiders. He hated that he was afraid and felt like he was less of a man because of it. He wasn't interested in looking at anything in therapy except his fear of spiders. In the beginning he told his family history briefly; overall, he'd had a good experience within his family and with other relationships. As we talked, I was looking for any events that might have led up to his fear of spiders. He couldn't remember anything specific, other than his current feelings. It is common with spider and snake phobias to have no actual experiences. With this in mind, we jumped right into doing preparatory work for his EMDR.

We started with his safe place. He was standing on top of a mountain with the sun shining and he could feel the strength of the mountain underneath him. He felt powerful and supported. He loved the feeling he got all over his body when he imagined his safe place and we added BLS with the pulsers to strengthen this feeling.

Next, he found his container, a big black box that he could put a chain around and lock with several locks. Finally, I guided him through a relaxation exercise, imagining a beautiful color streaming through his body from head to toe and letting the color melt any tension in his body and release any fears.

I asked Tyler again if he could remember any earlier time when he was afraid of spiders. He said that he could not remember a specific event but knew he had felt this since his teens. He said that he felt the activation of his fears rise if he even saw a plastic spider, a spider in a movie, a picture of a spider in a book, or even if people were just talking about them. All of these were clear triggers. We began to assess the first target in the list of his fears around spiders. I chose the first target to be an incident that Tyler felt had the most charge for him. There were no actual root memories or incidents that Tyler could remember that preceded any of his fearful images or triggers.

- Image: "A tarantula I saw at the museum."
- Negative belief: "I'm going to die."
- Positive belief: "I'm okay."
- VoC scale: "2."
- Emotions: "Scared and frightened."
- SUDS scale: "10."
- Location of body sensation: "Tingle and tightness of neck and top of shoulders."

We began the desensitization phase using the alternating tones through earphones as the BLS. Some strong emotions came up immediately. At times Tyler felt as if the feelings would be too much and the fear would overwhelm him. At the same time, he realized that he was okay in my office and could feel the feelings and move through them. He was surprised that by the end of the session he felt no disturbance. His positive belief had changed so that he and the spider could be in the same room and he would be all right.

We next looked at present-day triggers. He said he once saw a spider in his basement where he went to do laundry and he was afraid it could happen again. I had him find an image of this and connect to see if he felt any disturbance. He said he didn't, so we did a set of BLS just to make sure that nothing else would get activated. He still felt fine. We then proceeded to install his positive belief, "We can coexist and I'm okay." We went through every possible trigger he could think of around spiders.

Once all the triggers were processed, we moved on to a future rehearsal of seeing spiders in different places, seeing himself coexist with the spiders and feeling okay. We then added BLS to the images and the belief, strengthening the scenario. He felt no activation from these rehearsals. In fact, he felt good and no longer worried that he was going to feel fearful if he encountered a spider. Instead of reacting with phobic fear, he decided that he would to be able to find a way to get the spider on a piece of paper and release it in his backyard. We continued this process with all of his previous future fears until he felt confident that he would be okay in all the situations.

We completed this whole issue in two sessions. Tyler came in for his next session and reported that he didn't feel activated anymore when he thought of spiders. He said, "Let's see how it goes over time, because this change is hard to trust." Five months later Tyler called me to let me know he had encountered a spider in his basement and he was able to coexist with no fear response, catch the spider in a jar, and set the spider free. He also challenged himself to go back to the museum to see the spider that had so scared him before. He was thrilled that he could go up to the glass, say hi to the spider, and feel okay. Tyler reported that he no longer felt freaked out by such a little thing and that a little EMDR had gone a long way in changing his life.

Process Phobia: Robert

Robert, a 41-year-old married man with two children, came to me very upset because his fear of flying was affecting him and his family. He'd had no previous trouble flying until recently on a business trip he experienced a panic attack. He couldn't connect the panic to anything specific other than sitting on a plane. All of a sudden he couldn't breathe, his vision blurred, and he wanted to run and hide. He wanted this reaction to go away so that he'd be able to travel again and be okay.

He now had a job that did not require him to fly for business meetings. Robert had a steady job and a solid marriage, and he loved being a father to his children. His fears around flying were interfering with his family enjoying vacations. He felt fear just thinking about making plans for a trip and driving to the airport had become difficult. Even dropping someone off or picking someone up was problematic because of the phobia. Robert longed to be in charge of his life and not feel the fear control him and reduce his choices.

We knew that Robert's first panic occurred when he was flying, and that he had never experienced such a panic before in his life. It seemed clear as I listened to his family history that what he was most concerned about was his current fear of flying; if he chose, we could address other childhood issues later. For now, we needed to help Robert find a way to fly again.

We started with a safe place. Robert chose a meadow in a valley with green grass, which smelled fresh like after a spring rain, with trees surrounding the grassy area that provided him a sense of containment. We added BLS using eye movement to strengthen this image. At first he said it was relaxing but then he reported some black clouds came in that began to rain on his perfect place and ruin it. It's always important to have a safe place that feels good and peaceful. If something intrudes, I have clients let it go and find something better. Robert let go of his first scene to find another one. This time he came up with his room from childhood. He loved this room. When he thought of this place he relaxed and it was easy to add the BLS to support this restful feeling.

We then looked for a container. He liked imagining putting the fear and upset in my trash can and then taking it out to the dumpster, which had a huge lid. In his mind's eye I had him imagine this container and he said it worked great. He thought he might have to add a lock on it but he would see how it went.

For the initial target we chose the first time Robert remembered feeling pain while flying. I asked him to remember an earlier time when he felt this way, which revealed no earlier memory or root incident. The assessment of the target activated the disturbance.

- Image: "I'm in the middle seat and I'm trapped on this plane."
- Negative belief: "I'm going to die."
- Positive belief: "I'm alive and well."
- VoC scale: "1."
- Emotions: "Terrified."
- SUDS scale: "10."
- Location of body sensation: "Everywhere!"

As we started EMDR with this target, strong emotions arose. The panic increased and he feared for his safety. I checked in with him often to make sure he was grounded in his body and could process the emotion without dissociating—that is, leaving his emotional experience. He had strong somatic/body sensations that confused him, such as pain in his abdomen, constriction in his throat, and pain in his heart. I just kept normalizing them and encouraging him to go with it and trust the process. This intensity of sensations continued over a couple of sessions. At the end of an incomplete session, Robert used his containment and safe place skills. In the third EMDR session, Robert could remember the event without any disturbance. When we completed desensitizing his fear, his positive belief changed to "I'm strong and I'm okay." This was installed and he was happy to have this feeling.

This kind of phobia can have many pieces that are troubling for the client. We proceeded to look at all the parts of his fears: making the reservations, driving to the airport, going through security, waiting for the plane, hearing the plane start, taking off, landing, and then getting to his new destination. Again, this took several sessions to fully process. When he was done, he could see each piece of this phobia and feel "I'm strong and I'm okay." All the disturbance he felt was gone.

At this point, I had him do a mental rehearsal of flying in the future. Once he talked through all the details from beginning to end, I had him run the mental movie a couple of times with BLS. By the time we were done, he felt ready to tackle this fear.

We then talked about setting up a time when he would actually fly. He decided to fly to his parents' on his own for the first time without his family to test his new sense of confidence. He was nervous, but we had talked about his new strengths and how he would take care of himself if his anxiety arose. He made reservations and we continued to strengthen his resources with his plan. He was able to make his flight and felt proud of his success. He did experience some anxiety but accepted it while realizing that he was strong and could take care of himself and not allow the phobia to diminish his life.

As Robert continued to strengthen, he explored other fears in his life that seemed to be limiting him. Had the flying phobia not cleared, or recurred, it would be indicative of more underlying (and forgotten) trauma. Many times childhood traumatic events can be linked to process phobias and need to be thoroughly worked with through EMDR processing for a client to find peace in the present situation.

CHAPTER SIXTEEN

Performance Enhancement: Darrell

If you shoot for the stars and hit the moon, it's okay. But you've got to shoot for something. A lot of people don't even shoot.

Confucius

Over the years, I have developed a special interest in helping people realize their artistic and athletic potential by using a modified EMDR protocol. As a one-time professional dancer and currently an Argentinean tango enthusiast, I love seeing people move through blocks that keep them from achieving their goals. The basic underlying principles of EMDR are the same, but the protocol is slightly adjusted to support this enhancing process. The number of sessions for this procedure will vary according to the client's trauma history and how stable they are in their life. Remember, every individual is unique and treatment is determined by that uniqueness.

The protocol combines visualization techniques used by sports psychologists with a version of the work I do with trauma. I use this with athletes, musicians, dancers, public speakers, teachers, test takers, and those striving to become more assertive. For this work, it is important that the client already have a level of skill proficiency to draw on for resource development. This is not for the novice, but rather for anyone who has been successful in the past and wants to improve their sense of confidence and emotional control, and relieve any related anxiety.

Many studies in sports psychology show that mental visualization of an event can increase the level of performance. There are two theories about why this works: symbolic learning and psychoneuromuscular learning. Symbolic learning hypothesizes that when you imagine an activity, a coding process occurs in the brain. That is, when you perform in your mind, you lay down a template and code it into your nervous system. In this way the feel of a movement—say, a double axel—becomes symbolic, or familiar, to your body-mind. With repeated visualization the movement becomes more automatic and easier to accomplish when you call on your body to perform it physically.

The psychoneuromuscular theory hypothesizes that when you imagine a movement, you stimulate very small muscular contractions similar to those involved when you actually perform. The brain sends signals to the muscles to contract and the neurons fire to complete the movement sequence. An experiment by a Colorado psychologist, R. M. Suinn, charted the electrical activity of a downhill ski racer while he visualized his event. The racer's leg muscle contractions and neural firings corresponded exactly to the terrain of the course he was visualizing (Ungerleider, 1996). With the visualization you strengthen the neuronal firing so that the message from the brain travels to the muscles more efficiently and your performance becomes more automatic.

To show you how I combine this well-known sports psychology process with modified EMDR, let me tell you about Darrell, 28, an avid and skilled rock climber who came to see me after he had to take 2 years off because of knee surgery. He hadn't fallen; there was no climbing trauma. He had tripped during a hike and injured himself. With the help of physical therapy, after his accident he was again in great shape. But despite his strong will and best efforts, his confidence was shot. Repeatedly, his mind sabotaged his efforts during even moderate climbs. Negative self-talk had taken over and undermined Darrell's ability to trust that his body already knew how to climb. His confidence was shaken, and his fear had increased. He felt less capable of climbing and was becoming depressed. But Darrell wasn't interested in doing intensive talk psychotherapy. He just wanted to be able to climb again and enjoy his sport.

As I gathered Darrell's history, he reported that he hadn't experience much trauma in his life. We were able to move quickly into the preparation phase and establish his safe place and container. He imagined himself sitting on a rock by a creek for his safe place. His container was an imaginary box that he could bury in the ground and put a rock on top of. Darrell's level of stability and ease in using his safe place and container told me that he was already highly resourced and could handle EMDR.

Next we prepared to target the past trauma from his accident while hiking. From Darrell's description, this was when his troubles began. He finally had to give in to surgery to help relieve the pain but, determined not to let this problem keep him from doing things he enjoyed in his life, he followed a strict regimen of physical therapy to heal his body.

There seemed to be some traumatic stress reaction connected to the surgery, both before and after. This is not unusual. Before surgery Darrell remembered fearing that there'd be some permanent disability, and after surgery he worried that he wasn't recovering as quickly as he'd hoped.

We assessed Darrell's first target using the EMDR protocol: his accident on his hike and hurting his knee.

- Image: "Looking down and seeing my knee swollen and not being able to walk back to the car."

- Negative belief: "I'm weak."
- Positive belief: "I'm strong."
- VoC scale: "3."
- Emotions: "Angry and defeated."
- SUDS scale: "7."
- Location of body sensation: "Pain in my knee and tightness in my chest and throat."

We worked on desensitizing this target until it was fully processed and Darrell clearly was able to believe that he was strong. From there we continued to process all the surgery targets and anything else related that held some disturbance and could be impairing his performance.

Once that was complete, we moved on to performance enhancement for climbing. In this part of the installation phase I use a modified version of the protocol. I combine principles of sports psychology with bilateral stimulation to increase the strength of neural pathways. This is accomplished by installing past positive experiences and future rehearsals using BLS.

I asked Darrell to remember a time in the past when he was climbing and felt completely confident and good about himself. Again, he had no problem remembering such a time. He immediately recalled a successful climb when he'd felt great. We talked this through to make sure that it was truly a positive event and that he could remember the felt sense in his body as he danced up the wall of rock. I then asked him for a positive belief about himself when he thought of that climb. It was, "I'm in the flow and I know what to do." Next, I had him run a mental video of that climb three times from beginning to end, always keeping his positive self-belief in mind. As he did this, we reinforced his sense of competence and positive self-belief with BLS.

I then asked Darrell to focus on a future climb. As it happened, there was a climb coming up and he was nervous about it. We talked it through while he visualized this climb. I asked him to identify any negative things that might happen and how he would handle each of them. We also talked about what kinds of things he could say to himself at each stage of the climb, and how he wanted to feel. Then I had him make another mental video. This time I asked him to visualize the perfect climb while keeping in mind the positive self-belief, "I'm in the flow and I know what to do." I had him run this mental video in his head three times while reinforcing with BLS until the imaginary movie of the climb was completely successful.

Finally, I asked him to go back and run the mental video of his past successful experience three times, again with BLS, in order to connect him even more strongly to the symbolic or the psychoneuromuscular body-mind imprint of what he already knew how to do.

At this point, our work was complete. Now Darrell needed to go out into the world and test what he had just experienced. He went on a climb the next weekend and called to let me know the outcome. His confidence level was great, he said, even better than before his accident. He thoroughly enjoyed the experience and never worried about his confidence in climbing. His friends noticed the difference, too, commenting that he was climbing now better than ever.

Glossary of Terms

adaptive information processing (AIP). The theory that Dr. Shapiro developed to explain how EMDR reprocessing occurs. There is an innate neurological process that is jump-started by EMDR, allowing a person to move toward health. This internal system is intrinsic to everyone and memories are stored in memory networks linked through associations based on perception. When the processing of EMDR begins, the unprocessed information starts linking through the AIP and transforms all aspects of the memory.

bilateral stimulation (BLS). BLS is accomplished by moving the eyes from left to right, by tactile pulsers held in the hands, by audible sounds in each ear, or by hand taps on the left and right side of the body. BLS is used to facilitate the resource development installation, desensitization, and installation phases of EMDR. Also referred to as dual attention stimulation (DAS) in other texts.

containment. A technique taught as part of the preparation phase of EMDR therapy. It is utilized to strengthen the ability to handle upsetting or disturbing emotions that may arise during therapy or day-to-day life. It involves developing a mental picture of an imaginary container into which can be placed upsetting issues, emotions, or thoughts so that they will not interfere with a person's need to manage daily life. Learning to do this develops mastery over your emotional states and creates a sense of control and safety.

desensitization. The phase of the EMDR trauma protocol in which a traumatic memory is processed. Using bilateral stimulation to activate the adaptive information processing system inherent in the brain results in your brain being able to process the previously stuck memory. As this is happening, you and your therapist use the SUDS scale to assess if and how effectively you are processing the memory, and to what degree it is losing its disturbing charge.

fight, flight, or freeze. The three universal psychobiological responses to danger. Faced with what you perceive as a threat to your survival you will fight, flee, or freeze. A trauma response always involves one of these three.

post-traumatic stress disorder (PTSD). The *Diagnostic and Statistical Manual of Mental Disorders*, 4th ed. (*DSM-IV*) assists therapists in making a psychological diagnosis utilizing symptoms reported by a client. The manual includes criteria for PTSD and states that if a person has experienced or witnessed an event that he or she perceived as threatening, that person may develop PTSD. Note that it is the perception of the event that is the critical factor in the development of trauma. At the time of the traumatic event, a person experienced intense fear, or helplessness, or horror.

resouce development and installation (RDI). RDI is a procedure that helps clients strengthen any positive internal state necessary to help them face a challenging situation. This procedure combines imagery, mental rehearsals, and positive self-statements with bilateral stimulation. It is used to build coping skills that can be utilized in one's life and during EMDR therapy. RDI is frequently used to help a client prepare for EMDR.

set. The period of time a client focuses on a memory, image, or physical sensation while using bilateral stimulation. Some sets are long, some short. The length of a set will depend on how a client processes trauma and is very individual.

stop signal. When participating in an EMDR set, the client needs a stop signal to let the therapist know that he or she should stop the BLS. This signal can be as simple as lifting a finger. You will be encouraged to use your stop signal if you lose your focus or if you feel a need to check in with your therapist. A stop signal is helpful in establishing safety in an EMDR session.

subjective units of discomfort scale (SUDS). Developed by psychiatrist Joseph Wolpe, SUDS refers to the method you and your therapist use to determine the level of disturbing emotional discomfort or pain felt when working with a traumatic event. The scale runs from 0 to 10, where 0 equals no disturbance and 10 equals the greatest disturbance. Your therapist uses this scale at the beginning of an EMDR session to help both of you assess the intensity of your disturbing emotions, and then again throughout the session to gauge how effectively desensitization is working. The goal of EMDR is to reduce your SUDS level to as close to zero as possible.

target. The specific traumatic event or memory that is the focus of EMDR desensitization. A target consists of images of the event, the negative self-belief, emotions, and physical sensations evoked by remembering the event. A SUDS reading will show how disturbing this incident feels during the setup. Each traumatic event can include a number of separate and distinct targets.

trauma. In this book, trauma is any experience that you perceive as negative and that negatively impacts your present life. Trauma is often referred to as big-T trauma or little-t trauma.

big-T trauma refers to trauma caused by an event that you perceived as horrific, helpless to prevent, and threatening to either your survival or the survival of others. Shocking, dramatic, and intense, these are often life-and-death experiences such as combat, rape, sexual abuse, criminal violence, a sudden accident, a natural disaster, or an unexpected loss. It is this kind of trauma that often results in symptoms of PTSD.

little-t trauma refers to any event that happens to you that you are unable to process for any reason, whether the event seems large or small. Usually the event or experience leaves you feeling in distress and leads to symptoms that interfere in your life. The effects can be long lasting and distort your perceptions of your self and of the world, and may damage your self-confidence and your ability to engage positively and effectively in your daily life and your relationships.

trigger. Any external or internal stimulus that activates an as yet unprocessed trauma. A trigger evokes a body-mind response that is disturbing and distressful to the degree that individuals can feel the same physical sensations and experience the same thoughts and emotions as they did at the time the traumatic event occurred. Trigger stimuli are often subliminal, and sometimes unconscious (because the event has been forgotten), but when they occur they provoke traumatic symptoms that make a person feel as if the past is happening again in the present.

validity of cognition (VoC). Developed by Francine Shapiro, VoC refers to a measurement of how true positive cognition or belief feels. The measurement scale runs from 1 to 7, where 1 equals false (you do not believe the positive belief) and 7 equals true (you believe the positive belief without any doubt). One goal of EMDR is to increase your positive belief to a 7.

Resources Available on the Internet

If you'd like to learn more about the related issues of memory and the brain, or trauma and EMDR, here are a few resources I've chosen because I think that they're informative and not too technical (except, perhaps, for the peer-reviewed articles). Although some are older than others and I can't vouch for their accuracy, I can tell you that they all seem to me intelligent, reliable, and unbiased.

The Human Brain
The Franklin Institute Online
http://www.fi.edu/brain/stress.htm

Introduction to the Brain With Memory in Mind
PMI Memory Zine: The Source for Memory Health and Fitness
http://www.memoryzine.com/introductiontobrain.html

Remember This: Memory and the Brain
Suzanne Warren
From Serendip/Web Reports 1997: An article that reflects the research and thoughts of a student at the time it was written for a course at Bryn Mawr College.
http://serendip.brynmawr.edu/biology/b103/f97/projects97/Warren.html

Kids Health for Kids: Memory Matter
http://www.kidshealth.org/kid/health_problems/brain/
memory.html

Understanding Traumatic Events and PTSD
http://home.earthlink.net/~hopefull/about.htm

The Lasting Effects of Psychological Trauma on Memory and
the Hippocampus
J. Douglas Bremner, MD
Departments of Diagnostic Radiology and Psychiatry, Yale
University School of Medicine, Yale Psychiatric Institute,
and National Center for PTSD-VA Connecticut Healthcare
System
http://www.lawandpsychiatry.com/html/hippocampus.htm

Memories of Fear
How the Brain Stores and Retrieves Physiologic States, Feelings, Behaviors and Thoughts From Traumatic Events
Bruce D. Perry, MD, PhD
http://www.childtrauma.org/ctamaterials/memories.asp

EMDR Full-Text, Peer-Reviewed Articles
Nancy J. Smyth, PhD
http://www.socialwork.buffalo.edu/fas/smyth/Personal_Web/
EMDR/EMDR_Internet_Articles.htm

EMDR International Association
http: www.emdria.org/

Eye Movement Desensitization and Reprocessing (EMDR)
Therapy: Guide to Making an Informed Choice
http://www.helpguide.org/mental/emdr_therapy.htm

References

American Psychiatric Association. (1994). *Diagnostic and statistical manual of mental disorders* (4th ed.). Washington, DC: Author.

Baker, N., & McBride, B. (1991, August). *Clinical applications of EMDR in a law enforcement environment: Observations of the psychological service unit of the L.A. County Sheriff's Department.* Paper presented at the Police Psychology (Division 18, Police and Public Safety Subsection) mini-convention at the 99th annual meeting of the American Psychological Association, San Francisco.

Barrowcliff, A., Gray, N., Freeman, T., & MacCulloch, M. (2004). Eye-movements reduce the vividness, emotional valence and electrodermal arousal associated with negative autobiographical memories. *Journal of Forensic Psychiatry and Psychology, 12,* 325–345.

Bergmann, U. (1998). Speculations on the neurobiology of EMDR. *Traumatology, 4*(1), Article 2.

Blore, D. C. (1997a). Reflections on "a day when the whole world seemed to be darkened." *Changes: International Journal of Psychology and Psychiatry, 15,* 89–95.

Blore, D. C. (1997b). Use of EMDR to treat morbid jealousy: A case study. *British Journal of Nursing, 6,* 984–988.

Boudewyns, P. A., & Hyer, L. A. (1996). Eye movement desensitization and reprocessing (EMDR) as treatment for the post-traumatic stress disorder (PTSD). *Clinical Psychology and Psychotherapy, 3,* 185–195.

Carlson, J. G., Chemtob, C. M., Rusnak, K., & Hedlund, N. L. (1996). Eye movement desensitization and reprocessing (EMDR) as treatment for combat PTSD. *Psychotherapy, 33*(1), 104–113.

Carlson, J. G., Chemtob, C. M., Rusnak, K., Hedlund, N. L., & Muraoka, M. Y. (1998). Eye movement desensitization and reprocessing for combat related posttraumatic stress disorder. *Journal of Traumatic Stress, 11,* 3–24.

Chemtob, C. M., Nakashima, J., & Carlson, J. G. (2002). Brief treatment for elementary school children with disaster-related PTSD: A field study. *Journal of Clinical Psychology, 58,* 99–112.

Cocco, N., & Sharpe, L. (1993). An auditory variant of eye movement desensitization in a case of childhood posttraumatic stress disorder. *Journal of Behavior Therapy and Experimental Psychiatry, 24,* 373–377.

Crabbe, B. (1996, November). Can eye-movement therapy improve your riding? *Dressage Today,* 28–33.

Daniels, N., Lipke, H., Richardson, R., & Silver, S. (1992, October). *Vietnam veterans' treatment programs using eye movement desensitization and reprocessing.* Symposium presented at the annual meeting of the International Society for Traumatic Stress Studies, Los Angeles.

Datta, P. C., & Wallace, J. (1994, May). *Treatment of sexual traumas of sex offenders using eye movement desensitization and reprocessing.* Paper presented at the 11th annual symposium in forensic psychology, San Francisco.

Datta, P. C., & Wallace, J. (1996, November). *Enhancement of victim empathy along with reduction of anxiety and increase of positive cognition of sex offenders after treatment with EMDR.* Paper presented at the EMDR Special Interest Group at the annual convention of the Association of the Advancement of Behavior Therapy, New York.

Devilly, G. J., & Spence, S. H. (1999). The relative efficacy and treatment distress of EMDR and a cognitive behavioral trauma treatment protocol in the amelioration of post traumatic stress disorder. *Journal of Anxiety Disorders, 13,* 131–157.

Edmond, T., Rubin, A., & Wambach, K. G. (1999). The effectiveness of EMDR with adult female survivors of childhood sexual abuse. *Social Work Research, 23,* 103–116.

Foster, S., & Lendl, J. (1995). Eye movement desensitization and reprocessing: Initial applications for enhancing performance in athletes. *Journal of Applied Sport Psychology, 7*(Suppl.), 63.

Foster, S., & Lendl, J. (1996). Eye movement desensitization and reprocessing: Four cases of a new tool for executive coaching and restoring employee performance after setbacks. *Consulting Psychology Journal: Practice and Research, 48,* 155–161.

Foster, S., & Lendl, J. (in press). Peak performance EMDR: Adapting trauma treatment to positive psychology outcomes. *EMDRIA Newsletter: Special Edition.*

Greenwald, R. (1994). Applying eye movement desensitization and reprocessing (EMDR) to the treatment of traumatized children: Five case studies. *Anxiety Disorders Practice Journal, 1,* 83–97.

Greenwald, R. (1998). Eye movement desensitization and reprocessing (EMDR): New hope for children suffering from trauma and loss. *Clinical Child Psychology and Psychiatry, 3,* 279–287.

Greenwald, R. (1999). *Eye movement desensitization and reprocessing (EMDR) in child and adolescent psychotherapy.* New York: Jason Aronson.

Henry, S. L. (1996). Pathological gambling: Etiological considerations and treatment efficacy of eye movement desensitization/reprocessing. *Journal of Gambling Studies, 12,* 395–405.

Hyer, L. (1995). Use of EMDR in a "dementing" PTSD survivor. *Clinical Gerontologist, 16,* 70–73.

Ironson, G. I., Freund, B., Strauss, J. L., & Williams, J. (2002). A comparison of two treatments for traumatic stress: A community-based study of EMDR and prolonged exposure. *Journal of Clinical Psychology, 58,* 113–128.

Johnson, K. (1998). *Trauma in the lives of children.* Alemeda, CA: Hunter House.

Kleinknecht, R., & Morgan, M. P. (1992). Treatment of post-traumatic stress disorder with eye movement desensitization and reprocessing. *Journal of Behavior Therapy and Experimental Psychiatry, 23,* 43–50.

LeDoux, J. (1994). Emotion, memory and the brain. *Scientific American, 270,* 50–57.

Levin, P., Lazrov, S., & van der Kolk, B. (1999). What psychological testing and neuroimaging tell us about the treatment of posttraumatic stress disorder by eye movement desensitization and reprocessing. *Journal of Anxiety Disorders, 13,* 159–172.

Lipke, H. (2000). *EMDR and psychotherapy integration.* Boca Raton, FL: CRC Press.

Lipke, H., & Botkin, A. (1992). Brief case studies of eye movement desensitization and reprocessing with chronic post-traumatic stress disorder. *Psychotherapy, 29,* 591–595.

Loftus, E., & Ketcham, K. (1994). *The myth of repressed memory: False memories and allegations of sexual abuse.* New York: St. Martin's Griffin.

Lovett, J. (1999). *Small wonders: Healing childhood trauma with EMDR.* New York: Free Press.

Maquet, P., Peters, J. M., Aerts, J., Delfiore, G., Degueldre, C., Luxen, A., et al. (1996). Functional neuroanatomy of human rapid-eye movement, sleep and dreaming. *Nature, 383,* 163.

Marcus, S., Marquis, P., & Sakai, C. (1997). Controlled study of treatment of PTSD using EMDR in an HMO setting. *Psychotherapy, 34,* 307–315.

Maxfield, L., & Melnyk, W. T. (2000). Single session treatment of test anxiety with eye movement desensitization and reprocessing (EMDR). *International Journal of Stress Management, 7,* 87–101.

McCann, D. L. (1992). Post-traumatic stress disorder due to devastating burns overcome by a single session of eye movement desensitization. *Journal of Behavior Therapy and Experimental Psychiatry, 23,* 319–323.

McNally, V. J., & Solomon, R. M. (1999, February). The FBI's critical incident stress management program. *FBI Law Enforcement Bulletin,* 20–26.

Page, A. C., & Crino, R. D. (1993). Eye-movement desensitization: A simple treatment for post-traumatic stress disorder? *Australian and New Zealand Journal of Psychiatry, 27,* 288–293.

Parnell, L. (1999). *EMDR in the treatment of adults abused as children.* New York: Norton.

Parnell, L. (2007). *A therapist's guide to EMDR: Tools and techniques for successful treatment.* New York: Norton.

Pellicer, X. (1993). Eye movement desensitization treatment of a child's nightmares: A case report. *Journal of Behavior Therapy and Experimental Psychiatry, 24,* 73–75.

Power, K. G., McGoldrick, T., Brown, K., Buchanan, R., Sharp, D., Swanson, V., et al. (2002). A controlled comparison of eye movement desensitization and reprocessing versus exposure plus cognitive restructuring, versus waiting list in the treatment of posttraumatic stress disorder. *Journal of Clinical Psychology and Psychotherapy, 9,* 299–318.

Puffer, M. K., Greenwald, R., & Elrod, D. E. (1998). A single session EMDR study with twenty traumatized children and adolescents. *Traumatology, 3*(2).

Puk, G. (1991). Treating traumatic memories: A case report on the eye movement desensitization procedure. *Journal of Behavior Therapy and Experimental Psychiatry, 22,* 149–151.

Puk, G. (1992, May). *The use of eye movement desensitization and reprocessing in motor vehicle accident trauma.* Paper presented at the 8th annual meeting of the American College of Forensic Psychology, San Francisco.

Rothbaum, B. O. (1997). A controlled study of eye movement desensitization and reprocessing for posttraumatic stress disordered sexual assault victims. *Bulletin of the Menninger Clinic, 61,* 317–334.

Sapolsky, R. N. (1990). Hippocampal damage associated with prolonged glucocorticoid exposure in primates. *The Journal of Neuroscience, 10*(9), 2897–2902.

Scheck, M. M., Schaeffer, J. A., & Gillette, C. S. (1998). Brief psychological intervention with traumatized young women: The efficacy of eye movement desensitization and reprocessing. *Journal of Traumatic Stress, 11,* 25–44.

Shapiro, F. (1989a). Efficacy of the eye movement desensitization procedures in the treatment of traumatic memories. *Journal of Traumatic Stress Studies, 2,* 199–223.

Shapiro, F. (1989b). Eye movement desensitization: A new treatment for posttraumatic stress disorder. *Journal of Behavior Therapy and Experimental Psychiatry, 20,* 211–217.

Shapiro, F. (1991). Eye movement desensitization and reprocessing procedure: From EMD to EMDR: A new treatment model for anxiety and related traumata. *Behavior Therapist, 14,* 133–135.

Shapiro, F. (1994). Eye movement desensitization and reprocessing: A new treatment for anxiety and related trauma. In L. Hyer (Ed.), *Trauma victim: Theoretical and practical suggestions.* Muncie, IN: Accelerated Development.

Shapiro, F. (2001). *EMDR: Eye movement desensitization and reprocessing: Basic principles, protocols, and procedures.* New York: Guilford.

Shapiro, F., & Solomon, R. (1995). Eye movement desensitization and reprocessing: Neurocognitive information processing. In G. Everley & J. Mitchell (Eds.), *Critical incident stress management.* Elliot City, MD: Chevron.

Shapiro, F., Voglemann-Sine, S., & Sine, L. (1994). Eye movement desensitization and reprocessing: Treating trauma and substance abuse. *Journal of Psychoactive Drugs, 26,* 379–391.

Silver, S. M., Brooks, A., & Obenchain, J. (1995). Eye movement desensitization and reprocessing treatment of Vietnam war veterans with PTSD: Comparative effects with biofeedback and relaxation training. *Journal of Traumatic Stress, 8,* 337–342.

Solomon, R. M. (1994, June). *Eye movement desensitization and reprocessing and treatment of grief.* Paper presented at the 4th International Conference on Grief and Bereavement in Contemporary Society, Stockholm, Sweden.

Solomon, R. M. (1995, February). *Critical incident trauma: Lessons learned at Waco, Texas.* Paper presented at the Law Enforcement Psychology Conference, San Mateo, CA.

Solomon, R. M. (1998). Utilization of EMDR in crisis intervention. *Crisis Intervention, 4,* 239–246.

Solomon, R. M., & Kaufman, T. (1994, March). *Eye movement desensitization and reprocessing: An effective addition to critical incident treatment protocols.* Paper presented at the 14th annual meeting of Anxiety Disorders Association of America, Santa Monica, CA.

Stickgold, R. (2002). EMDR: A putative neurobiological mechanism of action. *Journal of Clinical Psychology, 58*(1), 61–75.

Taylor, S. E. (2000). UCLA researchers identify key biobehavioral pattern used by women to manage stress. *Science Daily*. Retrieved July 2007, from www.sciencedaily.com.

Thomas, R., & Gafner, G. (1993). PTSD in an elderly male: Treatment with eye movement desensitization and reprocessing (EMDR). *Clinical Gerontologist, 14*, 57–59.

Tinker, R. H., & Wilson, S. A. (1999). *Through the eyes of a child: EMDR with children*. New York: Norton.

Ungerleider, S. (1996). *Mental Training for Peak Performance*. Pennsylvania, Rodale Press, Inc.

van der Kolk, B. A. (1994). The body keeps the score: Memory and the evolving psycho-biology of posttraumatic stress. *Harvard Review of Psychiatry, 1*, 253–265.

van der Kolk, B., Burbridge, J., & Suzuki, J. (1997). The psychobiology of traumatic memory: Clinical implications of neuroimaging studies. *Annals of the New York Academy of Sciences, 821*, 99–113.

White, G. D. (1998). Trauma treatment training for Bosnian and Croatian mental health workers. *American Journal of Orthopsychiatry, 63*, 58–62.

Wilson, S. A., Becker, L. A., & Tinker, R. H. (1997). Fifteen-month follow-up of eye movement desensitization and reprocessing (EMDR) treatment for PTSD and psychological trauma. *Journal of Consulting and Clinical Psychology, 65*, 1047–1056.

Wilson, S., Tinker, R., Becker, L. A., Hofmann, A., & Cole, J. W. (2000, September). *EMDR treatment of phantom limb pain with brain imaging (MEG)*. Paper presented at the annual meeting of the EMDR International Association, Toronto.

Winson, J. (1985). *Brain and psyche: The biology of the unconscious*. New York: Doubleday/Anchor Press.

Wolpe, J., & Abrams, J. (1991). Post-traumatic stress disorder overcome by eye movement desensitization: A case report. *Journal of Behavior Therapy and Experimental Psychiatry, 22*, 39–43.

Young, W. (1995). EMDR: Its use in resolving the trauma caused by the loss of a war buddy. *American Journal of Psychotherapy, 49*, 282–291.

INDEX